SUPER
NATURAL
STRENGTH

Bob Whelan

To order more copies of this book please visit:

SuperNaturalStrength.com

Cataloging-in-Publication Data on file with the Library of Congress

ISBN-13: 978-1468083347
ISBN-10:1468083341

O'Faolain Patriot L L C - Management
c/o **Ellis & Company LLC**
20300 Seneca Meadows Parkway
Suite 200
Germantown MD 20876
bobwhelan@naturalstrength.com

Cover designed by Bob Whelan. Cover design
executed by Logoworks by H.P.

DEDICATION

This book is earnestly dedicated to a great physical culture pioneer:

Strongman Priest and Strength Coach
Father Bernard Lange of Notre Dame University

Whelan Strength Training uses many of the same principals of Father Lange's Gym. May this dedication help to keep his name alive before the eyes of our strength-loving brotherhood. We need men like him now more than ever.

ABOUT THE AUTHOR

Bob Whelan competed as a powerlifter for seven years and set several military powerlifting records, going undefeated for 3 years. He lifted natural and raw and had a bench press that was double his bodyweight, a deadlift that was triple his body weight, and a squat just a few pounds short of triple body weight. He squatted close to triple body weight for 2 reps in training.

Bob has a Master's Degree in Exercise Science and Health from George Mason University and a Master's Degree in Management from Troy University. He is a Certified Strength & Conditioning Specialist (NSCA) and is certified as a Physical Training Instructor by the International Combat Martial Arts Federation (ICMAF). Bob served as the District of Columbia National Strength & Conditioning Association (NSCA) State Director for over 5 years. He has been making Washington, DC, stronger since 1990 running Whelan Strength Training, one of the most comprehensive personal strength and conditioning programs in the world.

He formerly worked as an exercise physiologist at the National Aeronautics and Space Administration (NASA) and as the strength and conditioning coach at Catholic University. He taught a self-designed course, Strength Fitness, at Northern Virginia Community College. He has trained athletes from the NFL, NBA, NCAA, Women's Professional Basketball, and various combat and strength athletes. He was an off-season conditioning consultant to the Boston Celtics for two summers. He was the base varsity powerlifting coach and coached the team to the USAFE championship in 1983.

Bob is the (first) author and editor of the recent classic book IRON NATION - Passion for Hard Training and was a contributing author in the strength and fitness book, MAXIMIZE YOUR TRAINING. He was a long time columnist in HARDGAINER MAGAZINE, (Bob Whelan's Q & A), and had an article in nearly every issue of HG from 1994 to 2004. He has written over 100 published strength training articles that have appeared in other magazines, too, such as THE DINOSAUR FILES, MILO, HARD TRAINING, and THE IRON MASTER. Bob is the owner of NaturalStrength.com and the founder and coordinator of 6 Capital City Strength Clinics. Prior to making his passion his profession, Bob served 8 years in the U.S. Air Force and 5 years as a Federal Agent.

Bob is a graduate of the Connecticut School of Broadcasting and hosted a weekly talk show on WGTB (Georgetown University Radio). He is an avid sports fan and has an interest in the martial arts. He is also a published poet. In addition to his regular strength training and cardio, he spends several hours a week practicing close combat self-defense. He currently lives in Washington, DC.

PREFACE

Thank you for purchasing a copy of my book Super Natural Strength. Many of you may have read my first book, IRON NATION, (IronNation.com), but may not have realized that I have been writing articles since 1994. Super Natural Strength is a compilation of my best articles from Hardgainer Magazine from 1994 to 2004.

I'm very proud to have written for Hardgainer Magazine and consider it to be the best magazine in the history of physical culture. I believe that I wrote more original articles for Hardgainer Magazine than anyone but Stuart McRobert himself. I owe Stuart a lot for giving me the opportunity to write for his great magazine. I support all of his books and works and advise you to visit his website at HardGainer.com.

If you read each page with full attention, you will learn a lifetime of information about building drug-free muscle, strength and power. I have tirelessly fought against the use of anabolic steroids, and against the mainstream muscle mags (and training media) for pushing worthless supplements and training routines that do not work unless you are on drugs.

I've edited and updated some of the articles as needed as a lot of time has passed since they were originally written. In a few cases, my training philosophy might have slightly changed or I found a better way to explain something etc. For the most part, the edits are few and the articles are as originally written.

I have had a love for weight training and a desire to be strong since my earliest recollections. I believe my own training began around age 10. I have read every book, magazine, and course on the planet about this subject. I have also tried just about every program and routine and learned what works by doing it. I was training, competing, coaching and advising people on powerlifting and weight training, as a hobby, decades before WST got started. Even though I have a Master's Degree in Exercise Science, I freely admit that most of my knowledge comes from spending decades in the lifting trenches and not from books. Having the formal education in this subject is extremely helpful, however, as it gives my writing sharper teeth and more credibility to those not familiar with the culture of weight training.

Many Methods Work

How would I describe my training philosophy? Simple: First of all, never, ever use drugs to assist your training. Work hard, lift heavy, eat well and get enough recovery between workouts. In a nutshell, it's: Natural, Hard, Safe and Progressive.

Please don't read a few of my articles and think you know "how I train" or think that I train that exact way all the time. Remember that an article is a snapshot of one day or of one individual's workout. If an article has machines in it, it does not mean I always use machines or never use barbells. If an article is about using barbells, it does not mean I don't use machines. If I do sets to failure in an article, it does not mean that I always do sets to failure . . . and so forth. I always lift heavy, hard and focus on the basic movements. Make sure to eat well and get enough recovery too.

I view training modes and methods as tools in a tool shed. I use all the good tools in the shed. I use barbells, dumbbells, benches, power racks, good machines, odd objects, high reps, low reps, regular speed, and some slow speed. I focus on the basics and the compound movements, but many methods work and I use many methods. It all depends on the goal and circumstance of the individual being trained. Progression is the unifying factor that makes all successful strength training programs work. Keep an open mind about your training. Try new methods. Almost all modes and methods can work if you strive to lift safely and heavier.

You can keep track of what's new with me at NaturalStrength.com,

BobWhelan.com and NaturalStrength.net. Be sure to sign-up for our mailing list – it's free. Stay strong not only physically but mentally and spiritually as well.

Bob Whelan

ACKNOWLEDGMENTS

I would like to acknowledge the contributions of the following individuals to the development of this book:

1. Stuart McRobert

A tip of my cap and the biggest thank you go to Stuart. He is the founder, publisher, and editor of HARDGAINER, the greatest physical culture magazine in history.

2. Lorraine Maslow

Lorraine did all the typing and typesetting and helped me with the editing, too. Thanks, Lorraine!

3. Alan Leach

Alan helped with proofreading and editing and was a big supporter of this project. Thanks, Alan!

4. Osmo Kiiha

Osmo also helped with the proofreading. Thank you, Osmo!

5. Jewl Petteway

Thanks, Jewl, for doing such outstanding website work for me since 1999!

6. Randy Roach

Thank you, Randy, for all the great advice you gave me to help make this book possible.

7. My Mother

Thank you mom for all your love and support for 57 years. I love you.

CONTENTS

What is Life?

Is it just a span of existence
Or the number of breaths we take?
The accumulation of treasure…
or the money that we make?

Life to some means nothing
They throw their own away
But to most of us it's everything
but what? … we still can't say

To many, it's the future
They're constantly preparing
To others, it's the past
With dull eyes often staring

To me, life's an eternal second
With no future and no past
The awareness of existence
And the hope that it will last…

-- Bob Whelan

FOREWORD

By

Father Paul Makar

I am humbled to have the honor to be asked by a great man to write this foreword for what I know to be a great book. I not only consider myself humbled, but indeed blessed, for to know Bob Whelan is truly indeed a blessing. I do not say this lightly, nor to spout platitudes, but rather, I say this in thanksgiving, because "Maximum Bob" (as he is known to many) is a true teacher in the finest sense of the word. I have to say, some might see a picture of me and say, "What is that guy doing writing a foreword for a book on weightlifting? He can't bench or curl that much weight! Heck, he is not even strong enough to be worth listening to!!" Regarding the naysayers, I pay little attention to them, except to pray for them as they are too close-minded to even begin to appreciate what the iron game is all about. Such people cannot appreciate the saying that is printed on the t-shirts that Bob has made for devotees of Whelan Strength Training:

No Toning,
No Chrome,
No Bull.

Just the Workout Of Your Life!

It is a travesty not to appreciate this gem of a saying because when you are taught to work HARD the way Bob teaches, you begin to truly appreciate the value of hard work with the iron. It becomes not only a physical way of life, but it seeps into the mental and spiritual aspects of your life too. In metaphysical terms, it becomes a part of your very being, your very existence. This is a complete opposite of what is seen in the "chrome and mirrors" meat markets that most gyms are today, where the vast population is interested in scoping out members of the opposite sex, grunting and groaning to impress each other (that is if grunting and groaning happens to be allowed at that gym!), dance club Muzak blaring, and robotically going through mechanical routines (and sometimes shooting steroids) to look like the cover guy of the latest bodybuilding rag with overinflated pecs and biceps (or cover lady with the perfect legs and curves with only a hint of muscle – whatever the fashion rage may be).

I'll never forget when I first came across Bob. At that time, I was a simple, lowly seminarian studying philosophy and theology in Washington, DC, at the Catholic University of America. I was going through some tough times and happened to be looking up some information on old-time bodybuilders when I saw an advertisement for Whelan Strength Training. I remember being quite impressed at what I saw – the photos of people who worked out in Bob's "dungeon" located in the heart of the District of Columbia's Chinatown really captivated me. I especially was impressed by the photos of the many who tried to complete the farmer's walk around the block as a finisher, or those who wrestled the sandbag in the back alleys where Whelan Strength Training was located. I thought to myself, "Good Lord in Heaven, I want to be like one of those strong men/women! I am tired of being a fat body, tired of being depressed, tired of feeling run down by my thesis and course work. I need to change and do something NOW." It was that moment in life when a life-changing decision absolutely had to be made. And so I did something about it – I gave Bob a call.

I remember being very impressed when I initially called him on the telephone to inquire about training with him. We had talked at length for quite a while about what kind of goals I had wanted to achieve, where I had wanted to go, and what I expected out of weight training. This was something that I did not expect – here was a no-nonsense New Englander who took a very personal interest in my development and success from day one. This, I strongly believe, was the main indicator that I was dealing with a very special person.

I'll also never forget the first workout I had at Whelan Strength Training. If you are humble and honest with yourself and with Bob, he will give you the workout of your life. Then again, if you are cocky, arrogant, and think you know everything there is about the iron game, Bob will also give you the first (and probably last) workout of your life as well! I'll never forget the stories I have heard about macho dudes with big egos and lots of bravado coming into Whelan Strength Training thinking they can outdo "Maximum Bob," only to find themselves on the floor puking their guts out and lying in one flaccid heap of quivering, spasming, limp flesh, never to return again. However, if you got the right stuff and the right frame of mind, he will gently push and coax you to work at levels you never thought possible. Chances are you will be drained, soaking in sweat, breathing like a steam engine, and perhaps feeling nauseous. You will know that you have worked hard, and those workouts pay big dividends. During my time with him, I have developed my strength to a level that I never thought I had, even while I was on active duty in the U.S. Navy. However, there is something more important when training with Bob. He, as a true professional, works his hardest to draw the best out of every person he comes across. He not only sees the importance of physical training on the iron, but he draws out the mental and spiritual aspects of the iron game as well.

Being a Catholic priest in-training during that time, I had the unique ability to work with Bob and gain many insights from him. I, for one, never forgot my workouts with Bob. The first workout (and almost all of my subsequent workouts at WST) left me on the floor, drained, in a cold sweat. But there was something uplifting about it. Working out my hardest on squats, deadlifts or other exercises with Bob gave me a sense of accomplishment on one

hand, and a sense of serenity on the other. When I was in Bob's dungeon (I am always amazed at just how much iron and machines he packs into that small 3 room space!), all of my worries seemed to melt away – it was just me and the iron, with Bob to mentor me on my journey, and I almost always left with an intense rush with a pleasant feeling of euphoria that was coupled with the soreness of hard work. It was a feeling that told me that I was doing something good in caring for myself, and that I was showing God my personal gratitude for the gift of life I received from him.

As you can probably tell, my whole outlook on things is colored (or biased as some of my atheist/agnostic friends would say) by my spiritual upbringing in the Ukrainian Catholic Church. I see the human being, in his or her totality, as a gift from God. To me, this flows from scripture and from sacred tradition. Jesus Himself stated that the two greatest commandments from which the Law flowed was "You shall love your God with all your heart, all your mind, and all your soul. This is the first and greatest commandment. The second is that you shall love your neighbor as you love yourself." Now I am not here to make any theological commentaries on scripture and on Eastern Catholic tradition, but there is one thing clear to me here. I am commanded to love God with every ounce of my being, and I am commanded to love all brothers and sisters AS I LOVE MYSELF. Note the emphasis on AS I LOVE MYSELF. If I am to love my God and everyone I come into contact with, I have to be able to love myself. My life on earth is a gift from my creator. How can I possibly love God and my neighbor if I treat the gift I have received from my maker with contempt and indifference? Since I love my maker, and I want to reflect that love to others, I must take care of my own body and keep it healthy and in good working condition. I do this as an act of gratitude to my creator, to train it to be as strong and healthy as possible. It is an act of gratitude to those who know me and those whom I serve, for if I am not in good physical condition, then I cannot minister properly to others. My mental and spiritual health suffers when I am not in good physical condition. Ergo, not only is it necessary for me to train my body hard, but it is also an act of love – love of myself, for I care for myself, and love of my creator, for his gift in giving me my body and my very existence.

Physical training with weights also factors in something that the early Desert Fathers and later monastics used to preach about. (The Desert Fathers were a group of men–and a few women–who, in their zeal to follow God's commandments more perfectly and live a deeper spiritual life, left civilization into remote and inhospitable lands to live lives of extreme austerity.) A common theme amongst the many writings of the Desert Fathers and early monastics is the taming of passions. Passions, in the simplest sense, are those things that cause us to stumble, sin, and live immoral lives. They include gluttony, deviant and overindulgent sexual practices, greed, anger, listlessness, and so forth. These men and women went to great lengths of spiritual exercises to purge themselves of these passions in order to live more holy lives. Some of these exercises included prolonged periods of fasting, living under extreme conditions of poverty, and self-deprivation of sleep while chanting prayers and keeping vigils. While these appear to be extreme practices, the fundamental foundation is clear – to purge those immoral vices and passions from the person so that they may live truly holy and honest lives. They were truly spiritual warriors who trained their whole person – body, mind, and spirit.

In the same way, one who engages in the iron game must be prepared to engage their whole body, whole mind, and whole spirit when training. I know personally Bob likes to push each of his clients just to the edge, and then gently backs them off. When training, you must have your whole mind, body, and spirit engaged or forget it. I'll never forget how quickly I would be handling a very heavy weight that I did not even think possible until some unseemly thought or distraction would creep in and then BAM! End of set. Game over.

In addition, one needs to truly know themselves in order to get the most out of training. This is one aspect that I really thank Bob for, in helping me to critically look at myself and see where I am at so that way I could properly set my goals for myself. Now this was a part of seminary training – goal setting is very important to a seminarian and priest. It is no less important to the person stepping into the iron game. Without truly knowing your own limits and testing them, you will never, ever, reach the destination you want to go to. It is like traveling on a cross country road trip from Boston to San Diego without properly planning your route, reserving hotels, marking places and landmarks you want to see, etc. The journey will be miserable and you will miss many precious and memorable sights and experiences along the way. The mental aspect of the iron game is just as critical as the spiritual and physical aspect of it, and those who know Bob, know he stresses this important aspect.

The best thing about the iron game, and Bob brings this out of everyone he meets, is that no one is too young, too old, too fat, too skinny, too strong, or too weak to enter the iron game. The iron will meet you where you and your capabilities are at. This perhaps, I think, wrecks it for a great many people, who thing being strong implies being a steroid juiced junkie who lives 24/7 in a gym cranking out non-stop rep after rep as if there was nothing else to live for. Many feel intimidated going into a gym seeing all the hot spandex bunnies and super-ripped posers in front of the mirrors handling fancy colored dumbbells and grunting and groaning in the Smith machine. Some even think they will never get anywhere because they don't have the right genetics. I feel bad for those intimidated people for it is already game over for them. One should never feel intimidated by the weights. The iron is a tool which, through hard work, enables one to get stronger and attain better health. It matters not whether you can bench just a broomstick or 500 lbs, so long as you are doing something, you are well on the way to improved strength and health. Bob does his best to help you see what a wonderful tool the iron game is for any person. He is a professional who has the special gift of motivating you to work hard to attain YOUR personal best, to not be intimidated and try to be like the "Joneses" but to be YOURSELF and to be willing to endure on the journey to where YOU want to be. And that is what I love about Bob the most. To this day, I can still hear his voice in my head when I am away working out at the "chrome and mirrors" gyms doing squats or dead lifts: "Father Paul . . . YOU can do this! Get mad!! And, (sounding just like Kojak), REMEMBER . . . WHO LUVS YA?" To be honest, here in Philly, in the City of Brotherly love, I get fired up and motivated just thinking I am back at Whelan Strength Training and when I do, it makes me work that much harder. I remember all the people who I met at Whelan Strength Training and the accomplishments they have made and that motivates me all the more. I work hard and enjoy the results, especially the wondering glances from the people that seem to say via their facial expressions, "What the heck is this priest doing here?" Well, to those people I say that I am there for two reasons – to glorify God by caring for the gift of my body, and to improve my health. I am not there to impress anyone. True, I do not look like a model on the cover of a bodybuilding rag (and I don't want to look like some frankensteinian steroid monster – I just want to be ME, the way I was created to be.) I have a long way to go in achieving my goals, but my milestones are set so that way I get there little at a time. I have belief and devotion to God and that faith carries over in my training. There are many times I falter – I have my crosses to carry and issues that I currently wrestle with plus job responsibilities often distract me from working towards my goals. But, when all is said and done, the iron is there, waiting for me. Waiting for all of us to engage it to get to where we want to be.

In retrospect, I would have to say that Bob Whelan is truly a professional at what he does. I sorely miss working out with him, listening to the Patriot channel on XM radio during a workout (yes, we are no bleeding heart liberals here!), and getting all fired up and working hard, only to wind up on the ground in a cold puddle of sweat, gasping for air like a steam engine. On those days I worked out at WST, I truly felt a sense of accomplishment and when I would return to the seminary, I felt like God was truly by my side. Even my prayer time and worship felt so much better on days that I would work out.

I believe that God placed Bob in my life as one of my best friends and mentors in this world. He truly is a gift to the world and he is a master craftsman. I remember I promised him at the start, that when I one day would become a priest, I would bless his gym (I loved the picture of one priest who was a client of his doing wrist rollers in his collar). Well, several years later, I returned to make good on that promise. In the Ukrainian Catholic tradition, when a building is about to be constructed, or if it has not been properly blessed, there is a whole rite of blessing the facility, including anointing the walls/foundation with blessed oil as well as blessing the whole facility with holy water and prayers. Bob was so impressed that he said to me "God has chosen you for this Paul. You were meant to be a priest!" He is right – God has chosen me for this, but I will add that God chose Bob to do what he does. He was meant to be a professional trainer as well as a strong man. As I said before, Bob is a master craftsman, who is fully in his element when training someone and bringing out the best in them. There are some times in life when we have to decide whether or not to act on faith. I believe that when we do act on faith at critical moments in our lives, we are rewarded beyond our wildest expec-tations (even though there may be hard times involved). We all have watershed moments in our lives that demand we make a decision on faith and act on it. Mine was when I left my career as an engineer, sold my house and belongings and entered the seminary. Bob will tell you that his watershed moment was when he left a successful career at the CIA to make Whelan Strength Training become a reality. All of us, at some point or another, must make a decision on faith, and if we put our faith to the test, we find that God does reward us. In my case, I became a priest, and believe me, no paycheck on earth can match the intense feeling of joy when I work with people in my ministry, whether it is helping the homeless, holding the hand of a dying person who has no family or friends, or blessing a gym. In Bob's case, his reward is Whelan Strength Training and seeing people's dreams of good health and fitness become a reality. He truly lives his vocation every day and I believe those who have the good fortune of knowing him are truly blessed.

I will end this on the following note. I truly thank God for Bob Whelan for he is a true friend and a devoted mentor. One time, while working out at WST, I intended to thank Bob for everything that he did for me, but instead I blurted out in a funny way: "Thank you Bob for what you did to me!" Looking back on that now, I truly mean that wholeheartedly. What he did to me was to make me a stronger and healthier man, not just in a physical way, but in a mental and spiritual way as well. I encourage all of you to ponder on Bob's words in this book and let him teach you the iron game as he taught me.

Bob, in deepest thanks for what you did to me, I thank you and bless you. As we would say in the Ukrainian Catholic tradition: may God grant you and your family long life and many happy and healthy years - Сотвори Господа, і Многая і Благая Літа!

In Christ,
Father Paul
Philadelphia, 2011

INTRODUCTION

By
Randy Roach

Physical culture is about what you do in the dark. It's about how hard you train when there is no one to impress. It's about what you eat, how you think, and what you do on a daily basis. It's about doing the right thing.

The philosophy comes ahead of the end result. I don't care if they don't know anything and can't bench press an Olympic bar without any plates. That's not important. What's important is attitude. It's not how strong you are now, but where you are going that's important as far as attitude is concerned... They must be interested in doing the right thing.
--Bob Whelan

And just what is "the right thing" when it comes to true conditioning? Does anyone really possess the answer to this emotionally charged, commercially-loaded question? Bob Whelan is man enough to step forward and make his case within the pages of his latest publication, "SUPER *NATURAL* STRENGTH." To Bob, "the right thing" is simply the fortitude in conducting a training ethic that is natural, hard and progressive. In fact, "natural, hard, and progressive" would serve as a definitive motto for Whelan Strength Training. His T-shirts bear the words, "No Toning," "No Chrome," "No Bull," "Just The Workout of Your life" which also reflect the essence of this man's exercise constitution.

Bob has definitely built his own philosophy and sticks to it. He refers to himself as a coach over that of a personal trainer, the latter being a faction of the profession that he finds highly questionable. He feels that the vast majority of personal trainers have prostituted themselves due to lack of education, fundamentals, and a core philosophy. Whelan at heart is a pure strength coach. He does not believe in a fountain of youth, but feels that strength training is the closest thing to it. And Bob certainly has a set of strong core beliefs when it comes to strength development.

The readers are indebted to Stuart McRobert, the publisher of *Hardgainer*, a magazine from which the contents of this book were drawn. McRobert let a breath of fresh air enter the stuffy Iron Game hall in July of 1989 with the release of his first issue of *Hardgainer*. The compact, comparatively commercial-free publication steadfastly catered to the hardcore, natural men and women of iron for 15 years..

It was through the editorial craftsmanship of Stuart McRobert that Whelan was introduced to the *Hardgainer* audience in the September, 1994 issue. Stuart had cut and spliced a number of fax exchanges between he and Bob to compile an inaugural article titled, "Maximum Bob." From that point onward, Bob would compile his own material and be a constant contributor to *Hardgainer* until its finale in the spring of 2004. It was from that decade of contribution of articles and extensive Q&A columns, Maximum Bob Whelan brought a wealth of knowledge to the *Hardgainer* readership.

Although Bob holds a master's degree in exercise science and health from George Mason University and a master's degree in management from Troy University, academia alone could not give to Bob what he in turn shares with his fortunate clientele. What shines from his Iron Game soul he was born with and naturally cultivated on his own beginning as a youth. It was then that Bob mastered the heavy demands of pushups and pull-ups his father forced upon him.

Like so many die-hards of the game, he became hooked on training at a very young age. Bob continued with his pushups and chins, added cement blocks and copper tubing, dips between chairs, and everything else he could come up with until he attained his first York barbell set at the age of 13. With the York influence, he began purchasing *Muscular Development* and *Strength and Health*, followed later with *Iron Man* magazine. Bob captured the exuberance of so many youths that had both preceded and succeeded him through the decades:

> I was a fanatic and devoured everything related to training I could get my hands on. I was sad when I'd read all the articles in a new issue. I couldn't wait 'til the next month so I could ride my bike to the apothecary in Sherborn, Massachusetts, and buy the next issue. I can remember the smell of the ink in the new issues. I had to hide the magazines because my father thought all the bodybuilders were "musclebound," but I knew better. My biggest heroes were Bob Hoffman and, especially, John Grimek.

From these early publications, his fundamentals were cast. Bob was already mentally equipped to build strength and muscle with the most basic of equipment as demonstrated from 1976 to 1979 at a "small, dingy, minimally equipped gym" at Bitburg Airbase in Germany. He went on to both coach and compete for seven years as a natural powerlifter setting several military records on his way. His raw lifts are as impressive and extensive as the rest of his vast array of credentials too numerous to mention.

With such levels of education, depth of knowledge, and breadth of experience, Bob Whelan became one of our prominent modern day Physical Culturists: a hybrid of old and new. wise enough to endear the old, yet open to what the new era offered. He does not get stuck in the mud squabbling over pure traditions if common sense clearly shows that the old could benefit from the new. In his own words:

> I see myself as a tradesman with a shed full of tools... I
> see the various modes and methods of strength training
> as tools in a tool chest. A craftsman can collect and use
> many tools to perform his art. Only a fool would throw
> useful tools away and insist on using just a few tools.
> Different tools can be used for different people.

You will see this tradesman at work through the pages of "SUPER *NATURAL* STRENGTH" as Bob shares his arsenal of conditioning wisdom from the first installment of "Maximum Bob" in the fall of 1994 until the spring of 2004. For those 10 years, Bob remained loyal to the concepts of his trade with some minor evolution in areas where technology and further research had enlightened us all. However, you can't help but respect him even more when he uses his own experience, intellect, and common sense to draw the line on some of the modern day fads, gimmicks, and crazes that constantly sweep the fitness industry.

What you will get from these pages is serious tried and true strength and muscle building techniques and advice from one of the most passionate trainer/coaches in the world. Bob's mission is to bring the best out of everyone even if it means screaming encouragement at a young training enthusiast as he/she struggles to carry a 100 to 200 pound bag of sand around a building or simply accompanying a first time client for a gentle walk around the block. As hardcore as Bob is, that Military-based drill ethic is still governed by intellect and a rationale. As he says:

> Deaths are not good for business! ...A good coach must
> be a good judge of effort. Not everyone can give the
> same amount of effort. There are huge differences in

ability. Nonetheless, whatever they can give, I want it all. You must be smart enough to recognize the differences in individuals, and be a good judge of effort.... Extracting effort is an art form.... There are some coaches who don't think you've had a good workout unless you use the bucket. This is wrong. I view the bucket as getting a "purple heart" medal. You get a purple heart when you get wounded, but you don't want to get wounded.... You can't fake passion. You either have it, or you don't. If you've got it, it makes your job a lot easier, and a lot more fun. Everything flows from passion.

And it is passion that drives Whelan Strength Training. It was that same passion that led Bob to leave a lucrative job as a government agent, sleep only feet from the barbells of his burgeoning gym, and stay the course right to the top of the field. Passion ruled over silly arguments such as which was superior, free weights or machines. As Bob notes, "strength training is similar to religion as far as strong opinions go."

And with Bob, you will get in this book a solid philosophy on how to get the best from your body without drugs, powders, pills or any other magic potion outside of hard training and real natural foods. Much of the content of this publication is an extensive Q&A collection that spans many issues of *Hardgainer* from 2000 to 2004. Bob answers a myriad of questions including how to successfully build a personal coaching business plus much, much more.

I was both honoured and happy to write this introduction to Bob's book, "SUPER *NATURAL* STRENGTH." I agreed to do it out of gratitude for the years of work and effort he has put into his craft. So much of what constitutes Bob actually became manifest in his website, naturalstrength.com years before I had the privilege of meeting him. Naturalstrength.com was a godsend to me during my early years working on my own historical project. Only a man with true passion would put such effort and thousands of dollars personally into bringing so much of Physical Culture to the mainstream free of charge as Bob has done.

"SUPER *NATURAL* STRENGTH" is just the beginning of what will come to print from Bob Whelan's shed of tools. His first book, "Iron Nation," was an excellent compilation of training strategies from heavyweight players within the lifting industry. This second publication is "naturally" a compendium to his first. From what I understand and would expect, there is much more to come in the ensuing years from this super-charged, extremely positive, and highly motivating personality.

In the meantime, prepare to reap the benefits of a 10-year romp with Bob Whelan through Stuart McRobert's successful publication, *Hardgainer.* Bob will definitely take your training to the "Maximum!"

Randy Roach,
Author of "Muscle, Smoke & Mirrors"

MAXIMUM BOB

September 1994

I come from the old school of "health first, muscle second." I believe that if you can't get it the natural, healthy way, it's not worth getting. I practice what I preach and am not one of those 12-inch-arm academics. I am also not a "death-row convert" to the drug-free philosophy. Real champions *never* take drugs! I quit competitive powerlifting in 1983 because, even in the military, drugs were common.

I started a "personal training" business in 1990 and created a private gym in my studio apartment. My philosophy is basic exercises, hard work, and results. Business is booming. Real men want to work hard, but most "personal trainers" are the "toner" type. I have a sign over my "gym" door that says, "Maximum Bob, Proprietor of the World's Smallest World Class Gym." The layout has everything in its place like a Swiss army knife (only one client at a time can fit). I have a stairstepper, a rubber floor, no mirrors, no chrome, nine pieces of Jubinville-made (the best) heavy-duty black steel equipment, several York Olympic bars, and about 1,000 pounds of York (only) plates. I have slept on the floor between the equipment I plan to move to a roomier location soon.

Getting on the Right Track

Chris Hartman is one of my new clients. He looked like a walking skeleton when he arrived. He weighed 155 at 6-4! He was going to the gym 5-6 days per week and taking all sorts of exotic pills and powders, amino acids, etc. I had to twist his arm to get him to train only twice per week, and I had to twist it hard at first. But after the first workout he did not *want* to train more because he was so tired.

He threw away his exotic "miracle" potions and powders, and burned his former training instruction.

6

He now eats three knife-and-fork meals a day with three snacks in between. His daily nutrition includes five fruits and vegetables, one simple multiple-vitamin-mineral pill, and two cans of tuna (or turkey/chicken). He has gained 20 pounds already. He never realized he needed food, not BS from the health food store. He is now 6-4 and 175 pounds--a long way to go, but he is a believer.

ATTITUDE AND EFFORT: KEYS TO SUCCESS

May 1995

A few months ago a guy named Steve called me. He wanted to "tone up" and "body sculpt." I abhor those terms. He said, "I want to put on some bulk, but I don't want to get too big," (as if it were going to happen by accident). After he said "bulk," I told him that what he really meant was muscle. Bulk suggests something other than pure muscle (i.e., the bulking up and trimming down nonsense). He also wanted to "lift for definition." You lift to build muscle; period. You get definition by reducing your fat intake and doing cardiovascular exercise. (You must have muscle there already, or you will look like a typical runner.)

And here is the kicker: Steve did not feel he needed to work his legs. His were strong enough already, so he said. He said he could leg press 230 lbs (so can my grandmother). He did not want to do squats. He thought they were dangerous. He credited his "tremendous" leg strength to running and stair climbing. To my amazement, he still agreed to come by for the physical assessment, orientation and workout.

Steve sat attentively through the assessment and orientation, and seemed to agree with me on my nutritional information. When it came to the training, we had some problems. Steve—all 5-10 and 146 lbs of him—felt he was "too advanced" to train twice per week. He also felt too advanced to do only seven exercises for the whole body. He felt he needed several exercises for each body part. He wanted to infiltrate the workout with many little "toner" exercises, such as cable crossovers, tricep kickbacks, and lateral raises. He was incredulous that I could recommend only bench press (or incline press) for chest, only overhead press for shoulders, and only squats for legs. After I stated my case, and advised him that squats, properly performed, were not harmful but

8

could help *prevent* knee injuries, he grudgingly agreed to try the program.

Before we started the workout, I asked how he added poundage to the exercises in his previous routines. He seemed stunned, and had to collect his thoughts before answering. He stated that once he found the "comfortable" weight, he stayed with it and never added weight unless it felt ridiculously easy (which was not very often). Steve felt it was not important to add weight. He was "squeezing" and "feeling" comfortable poundages. He believed in long-term commitments and stable relationships with his poundages. He also did not know what was meant by working to "muscular failure."

After Steve warmed up for five minutes on the stairstepper, to elevate his core body temperature, he did a little stretching. Then, after I waited for him to adjust his sweatband, lifting gloves and wrist wraps, we began the workout. Normally, I start people slowly, but since Steve was so "advanced," we went right to it. After only five exercises, and one set of squats (with 125 lbs), Steve was too tired to continue. He said he'd never felt so tired, and didn't know "what was wrong."

"Nothing is wrong, Steve," I replied, "you have just been introduced to hard work. It's intensity with emphasis on progressive resistance—with the basic exercises—that are needed to get bigger and stronger. Stay with the nutritional plan, and rest. I'll see you in three days. If you're still sore, we'll wait until all the soreness is gone. You'll get used to it, and be amazed by the results you get."

But Steve wasn't interested in hard work. He was looking for some pseudo-scientific gimmick. He never came back. You have to put wood in the stove to get heat. There is no magic formula. High-intensity training, plus good nutrition and adequate recovery, is the combination that produces results.

I saw Steve the other day. He's still toning, shaping and sculpting away. He's still working his legs only by running. And he still weighs 146 lbs.

An Example of the Right Attitude

Contrast Steve's attitude with that of Alan Dinsmore, a client of mine who started a progressive training program more than a year ago. Alan was over fifty years of age when he started, but made no excuses for his age. He was not looking for gimmicks, had a great attitude, and realized that it was important to build a good foundation.

When starting with a client over fifty, you have to start slowly. Alan started very light. He didn't go all out for several months.

We focused on total fitness, which emphasizes cardiovascular exercise, stretching and nutrition, as well as strength training. Once you get over thirty, there is no excuse for not doing regular cardiovascular training. Cardiovascular work is just as important as strength training. Your goal is not to "look big" in your coffin. Cardiovascular training was done at least three times per week, and Alan worked up to 30-45 minutes per session at low to moderate levels of intensity. (Alan's age-adjusted maximum heart rate is 220 minus his age of 51, i.e., 169. The low to moderate, or 60% to 80% range, comes to 101-135 beats per minute.)

Alan's initial strength training program consisted of 2 sets each of the bench press, overhead press, row, and pulldown. Reps were kept high, i.e., 12-15. (But, after six months, reps were changed to 8-12 for the upper body and 10-20 for the lower body.) We added a little isolation arm work, did no deadlifts, and just did leg extension and leg curl for the legs. Squats replaced the leg extension and leg curl after a few months. After a few more months of getting used to the intensity of squats, Trap Bar deadlifts were added. Squats and deadlifts were then alternated and done once per week each (but never taken quite to total failure, for reasons of safety). We trained twice per week, whole body, with each workout lasting one hour.

For progression, we moved up 5 lbs whenever the rep goal for the set was done in perfect form in *both* the work sets (following warmups). These two work sets used what I call a "controlled" failure method. If you do less than the goal for the set, despite going all out, then you are going to muscular failure. If you reach the goal for the set, however, you stop at the goal. The aim is to get, for example, 12, 12, not 14, 6. On the final work set for each exercise, you go to muscular failure because you have nothing to hold back for. Do not change the sequence of your exercises during a training cycle, or your notes won't make sense.

Alan thrives on the hard work, and enjoys it. He realized that it takes effort to get results, and was more than willing to put forth that effort. Alan is about twenty years older than Steve, but is much bigger and stronger, and works harder. He now warms up with weights he used to "max out" with. After a year of training he gained nearly 4" on his chest, and nearly 2" on his arms. He reduced his bodyfat by 3% while increasing his body weight 4 lbs. He stuck to the plan, was willing to sweat, and got results the old-fashioned way—he earned it. And he trained for *total* fitness, not just cosmetic gains.

Alan is living proof that attitude and effort are the keys to success.

FOCUS YOUR TRAINING ENERGY

September 1995

To obtain maximum results from your training program, you must prioritize your training energy. Many people are simply moving equipment around and not using their energy productively. Simply burning calories will not produce muscular size and strength gains. Before every workout, you must first get your mind in gear to train. Secondly, *always* use good form. Don't expect a pat on the back for it; it is a given. Third, apply your focus and perfect form to *progression*.

Focus

The mental aspect of training is more important than any physical element. We have all read how important concentration and focus are to productive training. How many of us, however, have taken the time to really practice and apply it to our workouts consistently? That is one reason why I have no mirrors in my gym. If you train with proper focus, you will be too busy working to look at yourself. Look at yourself later.

If you are truly focused, you attack the equipment with viciousness. I have a sign on the wall that says, "Be here now!" Put everything not related to training out of your mind until the workout is over. The worst things to talk about during training are problems, as this puts you into a negative mental state. Everyone has their share of problems. Successful people have the ability to focus on what they are doing *now*. The problems will still be there for you to think about when the workout is over.

Training focus should be narrow, internal. I find that it helps to put a mental time limit on a "period of insanity." For example if you are doing a set of Trap Bar deadlifts, figure out how much time it

12

will take to perform the set in perfect form (let's say one minute). You now have a better mental target for your energy. Before doing the set, visualize yourself successfully completing the set in perfect form. Concentrate on going all out for the next minute, as if you have a gun to your head, as if you are on national television or, as I refer to it, as if you have put yourself in a temporarily insane state.

To maximize your physical potential, your mind must be singular of purpose, and focused like a laser beam. If your mind is split, you will never come close to doing your best. Remember this simple phrase: "If your mind is right, the weight feels light!" (If your mind is not right, the weight will be a bitch; but that doesn't rhyme.)

Form

We could also call this segment "Repology 101" as my friend Dan Riley, conditioning coach of the Washington Redskins, has coined this subject. The proper execution of the repetition is the single most important physical element in productive training. Intensity and progression will not yield maximum results unless they are performed with perfect form. Swinging around heavy weights will not produce results. Your muscles must control the weight without excessive momentum.

Few people use good form. Few people pause at the chest (with no bounce), keep their butt on the bench, and push the weight all the way to lockout when bench pressing. Few people go all the way down without swinging when curling. Good form, once you are past the beginner stage of training and are "potty trained," should be automatic. Doing a set to muscular failure does not give you the right to get sloppy with your form. You go to failure in *perfect* form. Any reps done in a sloppy fashion do not count. If one of my clients does a set of 20-rep squats and 5 of them were not to the maximum depth that is safe *for that person*, he only gets credit for 15 reps.

Lower the weights slowly and under control, and use as full a

range of motion as is safe for you. Many trainees routinely cut 3"
or so off their range of motion on almost every lift they do, under
the pretext of keeping constant tension on the muscles. If you use
toner techniques to work your muscles, then the weight is too light.
The resistance should be all that you can handle. Using the fullest
(but safe for you) range of motion is a classic rule of training, but
seems to have been forgotten by many. Do not go getting carried
away though and hyperextend or forcefully grind your joints at
lockouts. I am talking about regular basic exercises here, not rack
training where partial reps are productive and planned.

I think that using focus and good form is a matter of pride. You
can spot halfway across the gym people who know what they are
doing. It shows in their demeanor. Once you can apply focus and
form naturally, you can put all your energy into *progression*.

Progression

As all readers should know, progressive resistance is the key to
muscular gains. You should have a rep goal for every set, and
when you reach that goal, add weight. Keep detailed records of all
your workouts. Nothing should be haphazard. Get some small
discs and use them. They are truly "little gems," as Stuart calls
them.

It's the resistance that tears the muscle fibers and causes the micro
trauma that is needed for hypertrophy. If you go fishing and pull in
a 100-lb tuna, you need at least a 100-lb-test fishing line, or else it
will break. Pulling in that tuna, just once, proves that you have a
line that is strong enough. Your muscles are like millions of

microscopic fishing lines. When you use progressive resistance,
you force your body to repair itself, during recovery, as if you were
getting a thicker and stronger line. If you can pull in a heavy tuna,
you don't have to prove that the line can pull in goldfish. When
training for strength, you automatically increase your capacity for
muscular endurance. But when you train for muscular endurance

14

(toning) you don't increase your capacity for strength. (Toning is like fishing for goldfish. You can pull goldfish in all day, but the line is still weak and will snap when a bigger fish takes hold.) Your muscles will only grow as thick as needed to cope with the resistance you make them use.

Babe Ruth struck out 1,330 times, but he kept swinging the bat and hit 714 home runs. He did not let the strikeouts bother him. He kept swinging. People only remember the home runs. You will have many workouts where you cannot increase your poundages. But you don't quit. You keep at it. You learn about how to cycle your training intensity. You learn how to avoid going stale. You learn how and when to make changes that sustain motivation and progress.

Striving for progressive resistance over the long haul yields great long-term results. If you are working as hard and intelligently as you can, you will get your share of poundage increases. You may have to adjust your increments from pounds to ounces as the years go by, *but keep on striving.*

TRAINING THE OLD-FASHIONED WAY

January 1996

Downtown Washington was quiet and still dark as I walked through the Gallery Place Metro Station. My gym's front door was only about fifty feet away, in the heart of China Town. I arrived to open for an early morning training session with Vernon Veldekens. I've been training Vern for about eight months and he is about to achieve 300-400-500 status any day now. He is knocking on the door in all three lifts. He trained for a few years before I met him, so he was not a beginner when I took him on. For the last eight months he has been training at a new level of intensity, just what he was looking for.

Vern is the type of guy I especially love to train. He is a young (24) kid from Texas, 5'8", and now weighs a solid 195 lbs. He's a "throw-back" type not a sensitive nineties reader of a "fitness" magazine. He listens, loves to work hard, gives no excuses and takes no prisoners. He doesn't let minor aches and pains stop him. He eats endless cans of tuna and drinks gallons of skim milk. He does everything I tell him, without complaints or arguments. He spends far more time talking about his training poundages that he does his body-fat percentage. I like that. Guys who are more concerned with their body-fat percentage (when they are not fat) than they are with their training poundages have missed the boat. No matter what I dish out. Vern never complains and always comes back for more.

Vern arrived a few minutes after I did. "Yo Vern! Ready to kick some ass?" Vern's growl let me know he was ready. We started the warm-up routine. We'd both already had coffee and big breakfasts. Aerosmith was blasting out high-energy music and the atmosphere was good. We quickly forgot that it was 6 a.m. After he was fully warm and stretched, he began with inclines. After a warm-up set,

16

Vern banged out a set of 5 with 185 lbs using a 2 1/2"-thick bar. After incline presses he quickly moved to preacher curls using a custom 2"-thick EZ-curl bar made by Bob Hise of Mav-Rik. Vern willed his energy to get sets of 5 reps with 85 lbs. After a short rest it was over to front pulldowns with 155 lbs and Vern took it to failure.

Vern did three work sets for all three exercises. For the first two sets he used the controlled-failure method, stopping at the rep goal even if he could do more. On the third work set of each set he went all out to total failure and held nothing back.

After finishing the third set of pulldowns he was dripping with sweat. The black rubber floor looked like it had been raining and there was a hole in the ceiling. He took just enough rest to recover, but I did not let him waste time. We had a lot of work to do in a little over one hour.

I kept him busy doing a set of 20 reps in the good morning exercise while I changed some plates. We started the next round and I was screaming in his ear. "You're on national television! Hit the roof!" Vern pushed through three sets of 5 reps in the seated military press with 145 lbs using a 2 1/2"-thick bar. "Good work! You're moving up 5 lbs next time!" I shouted. He was breathing steam with piercing eyes. With good focus he headed across the room for pushdowns. Two sets of 5 with 95 lbs. On the third set Vern looked like he had been struck by lightning as his whole body shook and he went to failure doing 7 reps. "Moving up again, Vern."

Vern recently switched to a 5-rep routine after spending about six months building a solid foundation with 8-10 reps for upper body and 10-20 for legs. I believe in periodization or cycles, but don't want to have a long build-up period. We make a few minor changes and back down a little, but are back to full-force effort in a few weeks. I believe that *long* build-ups waste productive training time. In any event, Vern has been going like a rocket since I made the switch. We will ride this wave for as long as it will go. But I'll

17

make minor changes for mental purposes along the way. If he gets stuck on a particular poundage for several workouts, I'll take the pressure off by making a change, like using 5-3-1 instead of 3 sets of 5. There's always something you can do to get a mental edge.

Sometimes, when you're stuck at a certain poundage, the best thing to do is to *add* weight. If you miss it, you have nothing to lose and you can say that you got the feel of a heavier weight. But you might get it. In the mid seventies, when I was stationed at Castle AFB in California, I got 300 lbs for the first time on the bench. I remember I was stuck at 295 for months. I finally put on 305, had no pressure, and got it.

We were heading down the home stretch and Vern was slightly nauseous. I let him take a few extra minutes to rest and drink some water. "Are you okay, Vern?"

"Let's do it!" he replied. Next was seated cable row for 3 sets with 165 lbs, and then 3 sets of 5 reps in the squat with 325 lbs. I yelled in his ear so that he got the final reps in the last set. He got them, but collapsed after the last rep. I was about to call 911 but felt reassured when I remembered that Vern was only 24 years old. Some of my other clients would have been dead if I'd pushed them that hard. The nauseousness reappeared with a vengeance. I got the puke bucket. Puking is nothing to be proud of, but sometimes it happens to the best of us.

Vern was still keen, and the workout was not over. A little puking wasn't going to stop *him*. He felt better after a few minutes and said, "I feel good. Let's finish!" (My kind of guy.) He did some wrist rolling with a 2" pipe and a 15' rope that I hung over the balcony. Some people in the building were watching, and thought we were crazy. They simply can't believe that people *pay* me to do this to them.

After the wrist roller and a set with the Weaver stick, the final challenge is for Vern to transport a 200-lb sand bag around the building, keeping it at chest height. It's a bitch and even harder

18

than 20-rep squats. You can't believe how hard this is until you try it, especially at the end of a workout. Brooks Kubik advised me to add this to the routine about six months ago. At first I thought, "Yeah, right." But I decided to try it, and it was *brutal*.

I now have four 50-lb bags and can adjust the weight by putting them in a larger canvas duffel bag. The sand shifts and it is hard to grab. Your whole body struggles to grip, squeeze, balance and control the bag just to get it to chest level, bear-hug style. Vern had previously got 150 lbs and today he was going for 200. When anyone can get 200 around the building and *live*, they get a free workout and their names and date put on the bag, like the Stanley Cup. Vern collapsed about five times and it took him about ten minutes to get around the building. Each time he collapsed he had to wrestle the bag back in position in a sort of clean, which is no simple matter with 200 lbs. But he made it. But if I hadn't been yelling "Free workout!" he wouldn't have got it.

He made it around and collapsed. "Good work, Vern. Free workout. See you Saturday. Today, you built muscle the old-fashioned way. You *EARNED* it!"

Here's Vern's weekly training program:

Wednesday
>   1. Incline press
>   2. Preacher curl
>   3. Pulldown
>   4. Good morning
>   5. Overhead press
>   6. Pushdown
>   7. Seated cable row
>   8. Squat
>   9. Grip and sandbag work as time permits

Saturday
>   1. Bench press

2. Standing barbell curl
3. Pulldown
4. Leg press
5. Overhead press
6. Pushdown
7. Seated cable row
8. Trap Bar deadlift
9. Grip and sandbag work as time permits

Since we have the equipment to ourselves, and we have a time limit, I group the exercises and usually have Vern doing three different exercises in a row, taking about 30 seconds rest after each of the first two. Then he takes about 90 seconds rest after the final exercise in the group. This gives him about four minutes rest between repeat sets for the same exercise.

A workout lasts between 60 and 80 minutes, depending on if someone is scheduled after Vern. If no one is coming during the next hour, I hold Vern "hostage" for an extra 10-20 minutes for grip and sandbag work. Between workouts he does abdominal work, aerobic work and additional stretching.

WANT REAL RESULTS? JUST TRAIN FOR STRENGTH

March 1996

There are many people who just don't get it. I get letters and phone calls all the time from people looking for some kind of secret or "magic" program. They are usually looking in the wrong direction. Instead of asking how to make their programs harder, and get their poundages heavier, they are looking to get a better "pump," more "shape," and more "cuts." (It seems they have been reading too many "gentlemen's" magazines.) They make training more complicated than it really is.

Let me repeat: There is only one reason to train with weights—you lift to build muscular size and strength. Period. When you build muscular size and strength, you also get increased strength and thickness of bones, tendons, and ligaments. To do this, you must train progressively, using the heaviest poundages you can handle in perfect form in the basic exercises for the whole body. That's it! No magic, just hard work.

Most people don't want to hear about hard work. They will insist that there must be some hidden secret they are missing. If they would simply start lifting, stop talking, and put in several years of heavy and hard training, they would be amazed. Of course it is not easy, but nothing that is worthwhile ever is. To get good results you must pay your dues.

You will see some results after a few months, but what really counts is that you consistently train hard and heavy for the long haul. Heavy and hard training should become part of your lifestyle and be just as basic as brushing your teeth. Nothing to brag about, just a given fact. String several dedicated years together, focus on getting your whole body as strong as it can be, and then you'll see some *real* results.

The Pump

A good workout program is not determined by the pump you get. If you train hard and heavy, you may or may not get a good pump. A pump is not important. And it doesn't feel nearly as good as Arnold said it did. Any exercise with light weights can give you a pump. If you "flap your wings" with little dumbbells, your shoulders may get pumped, but they will not get bigger or stronger. After the pump wears off you will have done little more than burn calories. You must battle the iron, constantly trying to add more weight to the bar, or else you are wasting your time.

I know a guy who regularly misses his Tuesday workout but usually is there on Friday. He's there each Friday because he wants to "look pumped" for the women when at the bar later that evening. What a joke! He is wasting his time. The sad thing is, there are thousands of guys who think like him. They are lifting for the wrong reasons. They are only externally motivated and do not have the deep "intrinsic" burning desire for size and strength.

You must lift for yourself, not to impress others. If you do not have a strong desire and internal motivation, your chances to put forth the effort required are low. Those who do not have the necessary motivation for hard training are prime suckers for gimmicks, and are the reason why the gimmicks make up a billion dollar industry.

There are many people who think that "poundage doesn't matter" so long as you get a "good feel" from the weights. They spend their time "feeling and squeezing" comfortable poundages. BS! BS! BS! Get this in your head—*poundage matters big time!!!* If you want to be a "closet lifter," i.e., no one knows that you lift weights except you, then keep lifting comfortable poundages for a good feel, and keep "squeezing" till your heart's content. If you want to get big and strong, and have anyone who sees you know it, then focus on strength.

Definition

Cuts, or definition, is simply the lack of body-fat covering your muscles. Just because you have low body-fat does not mean that you will be defined. You must have muscle already built from heavy training. Otherwise, marathon runners and even Dick Gregory, Bobby Sands and all hunger strikers would have looked cut. You train with weights only to build the muscle. Your fat percentage has got nothing to do with strength training. You do not lift for cuts, or to get "ripped." This is a hoax and nothing more than exploiting the false theory of spot reduction.

High-rep strength training does not get you more cut. It is simply focused more on muscular endurance. Lower reps are focused on pure strength. This has nothing to do with the fat over the muscle, only the muscle *under the fat*.

Nutritional Factors

The primary method to reduce bodyfat is to add cardiovascular exercise to your strength training and reduce your caloric intake. Even protein and carbohydrate calories will be stored as fat if you take in more than you need.

To guide you in your nutrition program, never take the advice of someone who works in a health food store. Forget about the pills they recommend that are supposed to burn fat and get you ripped. They are a total waste of money. Health food store employees are usually the worst people to ask questions about nutrition. All they

are usually going to do is recite the manufacturer's hype to sell you all the "snake oil" that they can. People who work in health food stores are usually making close to minimum wage and do not have academic degrees in nutrition. Beware of the term "nutritionist." Although there are many legitimate professionals who use this term, there are also many "nutritionists" with no academic backgrounds in nutrition. The problem is that, in many states, there is no *legal* definition of this term, allowing anyone with only an "interest in nutrition" to call themselves "nutritionists."

For serious nutritional advice, only consult those who have the letters RD after their names (Registered Dietician). If you consult a dietician, find one who has experience working with athletes or high performance individuals. Then the dietician will understand your training demands. When I worked at NASA as an exercise physiologist, we had an excellent RD on the staff. I still use her, in her private practice, for my clients. If you need nutritional advice, it is worth the money to see a good RD.

When you do your strength training, you predominantly exercise fast-twitch muscle fibers, in the anaerobic energy system. These burn ATP/glycogen (carbohydrates). Your muscles and liver need to replenish their carbohydrate storage regularly because it can't be stored for long periods. It is imperative that you consume a high carbohydrate snack (300-400 calories) approximately two hours before your strength training session. Don't work out without being "fueled-up," or you will feel weak and "out of gas" when you train. Your muscles can't compensate for poor fuel.

Cardio/aerobic fitness training primarily burns fat as a fuel, and works the slow-twitch muscle fibers. It is not as critical to be "fueled-up" for your cardio training due to the constant availability of stored fat. (I'm talking about training for cardio fitness and fat burning, not a high-intensity marathon where you would need to carbo load.)

Remember, you only lift to build muscular size and strength, or you are wasting your time. The best way to build muscular size and strength is heavy and hard training, focusing on the basic exercises, with an equal emphasis on pushing and pulling for the *whole* body. You must pay your dues.

There are no secrets—just hard work, consistently done throughout the years.

IT'S HOW YOU TRAIN THAT
COUNTS!

May 1996

People are always asking me questions like these: "Which is better, 20-rep squats or 10-rep squats?" "Barbells or dumbbells?" "Machines or free weights?" "One set to failure, or multiple sets?" "Straight sets or pyramids?"

The answer is, "They all work!" We all have our preferences, but the *way* you choose to train (or the method) is not nearly as important as *how* you train. The key is that no matter what mode or method you use, you *work brutally hard*. You lift as hard and heavy as you possibly can—apply focus, form and progression. *Hard work* will make most methods work as long as you eat right and get plenty of recovery time.

You can loaf or use bad form using any method, and you will get poor results. You can have a negative attitude, lack concentration and just go through the motions using a Hammer Strength machine or a barbell. You can go for months or even years without progressive poundages using any method of training. Remember, there is only *one absolute rule* in strength training: high intensity training (hard work) + good nutrition + adequate recovery = results.

Everyone responds differently to various training methods. You should experiment to find the ones that work best for you. Keep a detailed training log and write everything in it pertaining to your training including how you feel, what you ate, any aches and pains, etc. Nothing should be haphazard. Review your notes often and learn from them.

The Basic Exercises

No matter what mode or method you use, you must include the basic exercises in your program. This is the foundation and does not change. To incorporate all training modalities—free weights, machines and manual resistance—I choose not to describe the basic exercises in free weights terms. Instead of saying "bench press" I'll say "horizontal push." Rowing would be a "horizontal pull," military press would be a "vertical push," pulldown would be "vertical pull." With this type of description it doesn't matter whether an overhead press is done with a Hammer machine, thick bar, regular bar, dumbbells or manual resistance. It would still be a "vertical push."

Many people do not have a balance of pushing and pulling exercises. This can contribute to joint problems. The musculature that surrounds a joint (prime movers and antagonists) should have balanced muscular development. If you spend too much time on the bench doing bench presses, and not enough time rowing, you are inviting shoulder problems. Overly developed anterior deltoids and underdeveloped medial and posterior deltoids will be the result.

When one side of a joint overpowers the other, it is almost like what happens to a car when the front end is out of alignment, and it pulls to one side. This especially applies during sudden movements such as playing sports. Many shoulder dislocations and other problems are caused by improper training and the imbalance of pushing and pulling.

The basic movements are: vertical push, vertical pull, horizontal push, horizontal pull, and leg-hip-back push/pull (usually the squat and Trap Bar deadlift). You can add a few isolation exercises, such as arm work, as long as you are not overtraining. If you are healthy and able, these movements should remain the framework of your program.

Intensity

There are many people who seem to think that "high intensity" only means "one set to failure." This is not true. High intensity, to me, means *hard work* and "one set to failure" is just *one way* that works for some people. High-intensity training is simply *hard* training. Intensity is defined by me as the amount of work done per unit of time.

There are four ways to increase intensity. (1) Progressive resistance—this is the top priority. The other three ways will do nothing more than burn calories unless you *always* include a form of poundage progression. (2) Sets to muscular failure, or "more reps" in a given set. When you reach the rep goal, add weight. (3) Reducing the rest between sets—get enough to recover but not too much. (4) Using stricter form to make the movement harder.

Any training mode or method that works falls under these categories in some form. They are all different ways of "overloading" your muscles, causing them to work harder than before. Many people argue that they have the *best* or *only* way to train. This is pure garbage. There are many methods that work, and thousands of people to prove it.

If you put an *extreme* emphasis on any of the four ways of increasing intensity, then there will be some trade off in the other areas. For example, if you put an *extreme* emphasis on minimum rest, then you will have to lower your base poundages. You'll have to do the same if you put *extreme* emphasis on form and thus do extremely slow movements. If you put an extreme emphasis on lifting the heaviest poundages, or demonstrating strength as Dr.

Ken puts it, then you'll need more rest. The key thing to remember is that we all have our own individual training beliefs based on personal trial and error, but there are many ways to build muscle and strength *if you work brutally hard* and always have some form of progression. In any successful program, using any method, your

27

primary focus is adding weight to the bar (or machine) in good form.

My Personal Training Methods

I'm 5'8" and weigh about 210 lbs at 41 years of age. I train my whole body on average twice per week, doing the basic movements with an equal emphasis on pushing and pulling. (Occasionally I add an extra day or two of rest between workouts.) I also do cardiovascular work, at least three times per week, for 30-45 minutes each time.

I do different exercises on each of the two weight-training days. I usually do low reps for upper body (5) and sometimes do singles. I usually do 3 work sets per exercise. My priority is to lift the heaviest poundages possible in perfect form. I put an emphasis on the eccentric or negative side of the lift, always lowering the bar slowly. I explode on the concentric or positive side of the contraction.

For the past year I've only used a 3" bar for the bench press and recently got 350 with it (with a delayed pause). I do overhead presses with a 2 1/2" bar and now use over 200 lbs for 5 reps. I use a 2" straight bar for curls. My Trap Bar deadlift, and squat, are well over 500 lbs.

I train in time cycles (not poundage cycles) and switch my program around after about four months, but always lift heavy. I

usually do 20-rep squats and high-rep deadlifts for one cycle per year, for a change. Although it works well for some people I don't like to do extremely slow movements full time, but only as a change of pace. I believe that many people who gravitate towards this do so to camouflage puny poundages.

Cycle Variation

There are many methods that work, and many ways to incorporate the basic movements, so why not mix things up a bit when you change cycles? This will prevent boredom, and maintain enthusiasm. I'll do 20-rep squats for four months and then may switch to 5-rep squats for the next four months. It's instinctive; my body usually tells me when it's time for a change.

Many people like to "mix it up" during every workout. This may be fine if you are very advanced and really know what you are doing. But I believe that most people, including all beginners and intermediate trainees, are better served by sticking in a training program for the duration of a cycle. This way you give the program time to work, and you really *know* what is working. If you change things too much your record keeping will be impossible to interpret.

Give you program 3-6 months to work for you. You will learn from your record keeping what changes to make for the next cycle. During a cycle, keep the exercise sequence and rest between sets constant, or your notes will be of no help.

My cycles are loosely defined and may go longer or shorter than four months, depending on progress being made. Here are three examples of cycles I have used, listing only the core movements and work sets.

Cycle 1

Day one
1. Bench press: 3 x 6-8
2. Front pulldown: 3 x 6-8
3. Military press: 3 x 6-8
4. Seated cable row: 3 x 6-8
5. Squat: 2 x 20

Day two
     1. Incline press: 3 x 6-8
     2. Behind-neck pulldown: 3 x 6-8
     3. Behind-neck press: 3 x 6-8
     4. Lying T-bar row: 3 x 6-8
     5. Trap Bar deadlift: 2 x 15

Cycle 2

Day one
     1. Dumbbell bench press: 3 x 8-10
     2. Chin: 3 x maximum reps
     3. Dumbbell press: 3 x 8-10
     4. Bent-over row: 3 x 6-8
     5. Squat: 3 x 8-10

Day two
     1. Incline dumbbell press: 3 x 8-10
     2. Pulldown: 3 x 8-10
     3. Military press: 3 x 8-10
     4. Seated cable row: 3 x 8-10
     5. Trap Bar deadlift: 2 x 8-10

Cycle 3

Day one
     1. Bench press: 3 x 5
     2. Front pulldown: 3 x 5
     3. Military press: 3 x 5
     4. Seated cable row: 3 x 5
     5. Squat: 3 x 5

Day two
   1. Incline press: 3 x 5
   2. Behind-neck pulldown: 3 x 5
   3. Behind-neck press: 3 x 5
   4. Lying T-bar row: 3 x 5
   5. Trap Bar deadlift: 3 x 5

Mental Toughness

You need mental toughness to make maximum gains in any program. I recently had a phone call from a 22-year-old trainee who said he was overtraining on 3 sets per week. I'm not joking. He needs a serious attitude adjustment. Don't overtrain, *but do train.* Many people are more concerned about overtraining than they are about training. If you stick to the basic movements, training only twice per week, and only squatting and deadlifting once a week each, you should have plenty of recovery. You must pay your dues.

Be tough and train hard. I strongly recommend that you order *The Psychology of Winning* by Dennis Waitley. Also order *The Magic of Thinking Big* by David Schwartz at your bookstore.

True Dedication

Many people talk a good game but are not really dedicated. Do you drink alcohol? If so, how many days per week? This is a weak link for many. If you are pounding beers more than one night per week, I question your dedication. If you use *any* tobacco products, you're not dedicated. Junk food? Sleep? Cardiovascular exercise? Mental focus? Find your weak link and work on it.

No Magic Formula

The same rules apply to all the modes and methods of training previously mentioned. Try them out and find the one(s) that work for you. There is more than one way to get great results. Beware of "research" and statistics that claim one method to be superior. Disraeli once said, "There are three kinds of lies: lies, damned lies, and statistics." If you look closely there is usually something being sold. Every camp that espouses a certain "superiority theory" has their own pet researcher. This is one of the reasons why the training field is so confusing for beginners.

Stick to the basic training philosophy, no matter which training method you use. Remember, the method is not nearly as important as *how* you train. You can succeed using any of the methods mentioned in this article, if you are totally committed and *work your whole body brutally hard*, eat right, have a positive attitude, and get plenty of recovery.

Authors Update: One set to failure is the most TIME EFFICIENT way to train, but you do not need to train to failure to get great results. It all depends on YOU GOAL. As long as you lift heavy and progressive you will get great results. If you do one set to failure with light weight, it is no better than body weight exercise and ceases to be strength training.

THE CAMARADERIE OF EFFORT

July 1996

"There is something in good men that really yearns for discipline and the harsh reality of head to head combat...I firmly believe that any man's finest hour, his greatest fulfillment to all he holds dear, is that moment when he has to work his heart out in a good cause and he's exhausted on the field of battle—victorious!"
—Vince Lombardi

Matt Brown was lying on the hallway floor, semi-conscious and breathing like a steam engine, with the 200-lb sandbag in front of him. A month ago he got 150 but 200 is a whole new animal. He had just collapsed for the final time today, while trying to get the

bag all the way around the perimeter hallways of the building. And this was after a grueling one-hour high-intensity workout. There was nothing left. KOed. Comatose. Workout finished.

There are only four names on the bag and Matt is not *yet* one of them, but he always gives it his all and earns the respect of anyone who watches him train and hears the noise he makes. He usually manages to go an extra few steps with the bag each time he tries it. It's only a matter of time before he gets it all the way around the building, and his name on the bag. Matt has gained 20 lbs of muscle this past year and his bodyfat has gone down. Six months ago, the 100-lb bag put him down for the count.

Effort, Not Just Poundage, earns respect

The key thing to remember is that it is not just how much weight you lift that earns the respect of yourself and others. It's how hard you work. You can't fake all-out effort. If you are not going all out, you will get less respect and not feel as good about yourself, no matter what poundage you are lifting. I know some strong powerlifters who have not broken a sweat in years! They are strong and worked hard (years ago) to build their strength, but for the last few years have been coasting. I'm not criticizing all powerlifters, but a lot of lifters could be even stronger if they continued to work hard and not "get satisfied" with a moderate level of strength.

There is something about the camaraderie of effort that brings about respect and goodwill. Too bad that they don't give Nobel peace prizes to places like the few good old-fashioned gyms. The good gyms do more to bring about brotherhood and camaraderie than all the theorists, philosophers and politicians combined. At the good gyms like Iron Island Gym and The Pit, they appreciate hard work and will root for you when you are going for a personal record. It doesn't matter what the poundage is. If it's a PR, it's something to root for. It's effort that gets respect, and the maximization of your genetic physical potential. And it's not what you've done in the past that counts, but what you're doing now.

Vern Veldekens was scheduled after Matt, and arrived a few minutes early. He was rooting Matt on during his last set of Trap Bar deadlifts and his battle with the sandbag. You cant help but root for, respect, and like a guy who works his guts out. Matt went several steps farther than he thought possible due to the encouragement and friendly peer pressure (i.e., screaming) of Vern, myself and other patrons of the third floor who are getting used to this, and enjoy watching.

An hour later, Vern would end up in the same shape as Matt, except today he would not even make it to the sandbag. I made him do his Trap Bar deadlifts *Iron Island Gym* style. He went to what *most people* would call muscular failure, at about 15 reps, *then managed to get 5 more reps*, with each rep being a life or death effort. At 20, he collapsed. I then let him rest for one minute (timed), but did not let him take his hands off the handles of the bar. He had to rest in a squatting position and just suck in as much air as possible. At one minute it was *go again!* All out to failure. KOed! Workout *over!* My "Iron Brother," Drew (the human wall) Israel, passed on this torture technique when he stopped by for a visit recently.

Drew and I had a great time "killing" each other. After our workout was over I made the mistake of trying to keep up with Drew with a knife and fork. Dr. Ken called earlier that day to warn me: "Keep your hands off the table when eating with Drew because he might stick his fork into them!" That boy can *eat!* It was Thanksgiving three times over.

Drew leaves camaraderie-building messages on my answering machine, such as, "Kick Vern's ass today, Bob. I want him on the floor." Vern replies, "Thanks, Drew. I love you, man!"

When I first met Vern, over one year ago, I didn't like him at first. He came into the gym with a baseball cap on backwards, which I didn't like and wrongly perceived as disrespect. I didn't smile or say a nice word to him, and was like a drill sergeant. He called me "Sir." I really busted his ass extra hard. Vern took whatever I threw at him with no complaints. After a few workouts I totally changed my mind about him and he earned my respect. We laugh about this now. You can't help but like a guy who gives it his all.

It's the same for women. Muscle tissue is not defined as male or female, but only as *human*, and will respond to hard training regardless of gender. With any *individual* you start with whatever can be handled and build up from there. No one at my gym works harder than Charlene McNamara. I train her the same as a guy. No BS toning. She said, in the past, she was getting *so sick of being "babied"* because she was a woman. She loves training hard, and ends up on the floor after many workouts. She recently carried around the building a barrel filled with sand that weighs more than she does, and after a brutal one-hour workout. She now has her name on the barrel in large mailbox letters for all to see. She is respected by all because she works her ass off!

Gym Atmosphere

The training atmosphere of a gym is far more important than the equipment in it. Some gyms have great equipment but a dead atmosphere. No one is working, and no banging, shouting, grunting and groaning are allowed. No camaraderie. Soon there will be gyms filled with great equipment but there will be no sweating allowed! These are toner gyms. If you are in one, find another gym.

I had some of the best workouts of my life at a poorly-equipped and crowded gym at an Air Base in Germany—rusty weights, creaky floors, broken cables, etc. But boy, what a great atmosphere! Several hard workers were always in there. Weights were banging, sweat was dripping, people were screaming, and chalk was everywhere. Just the basic Olympic bars and plates, a flat bench, and a squat rack was all we really needed.

Willie Bell the powerlifter, and Glenn Pieschke (former Mr. YMCA USA) were stationed there, with a lot of other strong good guys. I made great gains there. The gym was a dump but what atmosphere and camaraderie! We were all friends and had a great time training together.

Compete Against Yourself

Put for the effort to compete against yourself, not others. You never lose when you compete against yourself. Don't get overly concerned with numbers, but always be concerned with progression. As long as you are striving to add weight to the bar and giving an all-out effort, you will never be criticized. You will be respected. People respect *effort*. You should feel good about yourself. If you consistently put forth the effort, the numbers will keep going up.

Don't get discouraged. Keep striving! Nothing in life that is worthwhile is easy. If it was easy, then every wimp in the world would be strong and that would take all the fun and camaraderie out of training.

TOTAL COMMITMENT
REQUIRED

September 1996

"A change in the body can cause a change in the soul."
—Aristotle

The other day I was walking past a local downtown gym and couldn't believe my eyes! There was a guy coming out of the door just after working out, and he was lighting up a cigarette. I felt like punching him because it was so sacrilegious. It was obvious that this guy has no commitment, does not care about health, and is training for the wrong reasons, with only mere cosmetic goals.

Physical culture is about what you do in the dark. It's about how hard you train when there is no one to impress. It's about what you eat, how you think, and what you do on a daily basis. It's about doing the right thing.

I talk to guys all the time who say that they can't gain weight. Most are wasting their money on every type of powder, pill and "magic" potion, but don't have enough discipline and common sense to have a big breakfast every day. Some tell me "how hard" they train and they can't understand why they are getting nowhere. However, some of them neglect to tell me that they are out till 2 AM two or three nights per week drinking beer. (I find out about this sooner or later.) Some complain that they can't reduce their bodyfat no matter what they do. Their genetics are bad, they say, or their "metabolism is too low." But they are only doing cardiovascular exercise once or twice a week, if at all.

Unless you are a *competitive strength athlete*, e.g., shot putter or discus thrower, three times per week is the *minimum* for CV work. If you have a lot of extra fat you should be doing CV work four or five days per week. The duration for the CV work should be at least 20 minutes at target heart rate, or 30 minutes of total time as the warmup and cooldown parts don't count. And at least 30 minutes of target heart rate work would be wise for most. You can train for shorter duration if you do an interval style higher intensity workout.

There is a lot of nonsense in "muscle magazines" about strength training, nutrition and cardiovascular exercise. Just because a drug-using bodybuilder with no academic background in exercise or nutrition writes that he trains with weights three hours per day, six days per week, and does CV training twice per week, does that mean that you should also train incorrectly?

Before accepting information as fact, check the source. If you want to be put in a coffin *sooner*, then follow some of the ridiculous diets that are currently in style. Scrutinize any nutritional advice not given by a Registered Dietician, and don't easily accept anything as fact. Anything that sounds suspicious you must get checked out by a good Registered Dietician who works with athletes and understands their nutritional demands. Nancy Clark is an example of the sort of Registered Dietician I mean.

Commitment is about self-control, self-respect, hard work, and a desire for the truth, not the latest trend. Commitment is trying to do the right thing all the time. You do it for yourself, not to impress others. It is a way of life or a sacred belief. Total lifestyle commitment is what it takes to maximize your potential. It's not training only for cosmetics where the end justifies the means. If you focus on doing the right thing and making the right choices, every day, cosmetic results *as well as* good health and muscular strength will be yours.

A few years ago, while attending a sports psychology conference at the University of Virginia, I picked up a copy of that university's football conditioning program. There was a quote in there that I loved, and I put on the wall of my gym:

Pride

38

The best kind of pride
is that which compels you
to do your best
even if no one else is watching.

When people call me about training I can tell right away if they are serious. They must be interested in *doing the right thing.* The philosophy comes *ahead* of the end result. I don't care if they don't know anything and can't bench press an Olympic bar without any plates. That's not important. What's important is attitude. It's not how strong you are now, but *where you are going* that's important as far as attitude is concerned. If they have a good attitude, will listen (not talk), are willing to work hard, and are not looking for gimmicks, we will get along just fine. But if they argue, and are only concerned with attaining a certain look, they're gone. I call it the "phone test."

Over the phone I ask several lifestyle questions, and if they are not answered properly, then it's, "Take a hike, pal, call someone else. Don't waste my time." Many people talk a good game but when it gets down to details they are not really dedicated. If they smoke (or use any type of tobacco product), use steroids or any drugs, abuse alcohol, don't do cardiovascular training or stretching, and if their primary reason for training is cosmetic, not functional, they are nothing but phonies. I actually have my own version of The Ten Commandments complete with "Thou shalts" and "Thou shalt nots." They must be followed. I'm not just looking for clients, but physical culture disciples. There is a big difference. I want *true believers.*

Lack of true belief in a program, or lack of a training philosophy, is one of the biggest problems with most so-called "personal trainers." There are some good "personal trainers," but the vast majority are unqualified, uncommitted leeches who say anything to steal your money. I'm embarrassed to call myself a personal trainer. I'm a coach. Most personal trainers will do what *you* want and say what *you* want to hear, to get your money. I believe that most personal trainers are nothing more than "fitness prostitutes."

A coach has a philosophy and sticks to this philosophy regardless if you sign up as a client or not.

Toning and shaping, and similar words, are swear words in my program. You train only for strength. If you consistently train hard, heavy and correctly you will reap your just share of cosmetic results. But it's not the focus. You don't dwell on it. You dwell on training hard. You get hat you earn.

If you are interviewed for a job, you don't ask about when you are going to get paid, or talk about how you are going to spend your money. You talk about doing a good job. That's how you will get hired. Focus on doing a good job; the pay comes later. It's the same principle with strength training.

The Nutritional Factor

If you are trying to gain muscular weight, you *must* eat a big breakfast every day. No excuses! Nutrition is about absorption. We already lose about 12 hours per day of our potential daily nutrition—between dinner and breakfast, from about 6 PM to 6 AM depending on the individual. That is *if you eat breakfast*. If you don't eat breakfast, you may spend as much as 18 hours out of every 24 with no nutrition.

What law says you must have cereal for breakfast? I know some high-caliber athletes who eat chicken, vegetables, salad, potatoes, etc., for breakfast. Who says that you can't? Champions look to find an edge. Champions don't want to be normal. Have you ever thought of setting your alarm for 2 AM and getting up for an extra meal? Most "normal" people would never do that. A champion will do it.

For lunch, do you regularly eat sandwiches or do you eat a big knife-and-fork type meal? For most people it wouldn't matter, but if you are trying to gain muscle it could make all the difference. A cafeteria-style knife-and-fork type meal with salad, vegetables, potatoes or rice, and meat, fish or chicken is far more beneficial for gaining muscle than is a simple sandwich-type lunch. You need 5-9 portions of fruits and vegetables per day. It's hard to fit that bill by wasting a meal on sandwiches. Use sandwiches as your snacks between meals.

If you are trying to gain muscle, do you eat two cans of tuna packed in water per day in between your meals? Not as meals but *in between* them. If you are dedicated and committed you'll do it. You can use chicken or turkey if you get sick of tuna. You could drink half a gallon of *skim* milk per day instead of the tuna in between meals. Don't waste your money on powders and amino acids. You don't need them, but you will still get plenty of protein simply by using the natural supplement of regular food as I have just described. You will not only be getting enough protein, you will *be wasting* a lot.

Have you ever made an appointment with a good Registered Dietician? Most people don't do it and amazingly would never even think of it. But yet they will trust their nutritional health to a minimum-wage clerk who works in the health food store, or a drug-using bodybuilder.

Many People Are Afraid to Succeed

Many people are not willing to go the extra mile because they don't want to stand out. They feel more comfortable blending in with the crowd. I tell people, "You don't want to be *normal*. You want to be far better than that." You should think of things to do that most "normal" people don't do. Unusual dedication is not normal, but is required to maximize your potential.

Obviously you should not overtrain, and the mega-hype routines don't work for non-drug users. However, two hard workouts per week or two hard workouts per nine days should provide sufficient rest. Do you spend more time talking about *overtraining* and not enough time *training?* This is a common problem these days. Many people have no idea what a hard workout is like and at the slightest bit of fatigue or discomfort will quit. Incredibly, many

41

underachievers claim to need 7-10 days between their workout days when they are really ready following three or four days of rest. Their muscles have begun to atrophy by the time they do their next workout.

Injuries are a serious subject and I don't mean to downplay this. There is a difference, however, between a rational concern for safety and a fear or paranoia concerning injuries. This is a mental toughness issue. A sharp pain is an injury and should be medically checked out. A dull muscular ache is normal. It's part of training hard. Many will consider the slightest minor ache to be an injury and use it as an excuse to take a few weeks off. The truth is that many of these people have a deep dislike for hard training but won't admit it.

Do you religiously train hard or do you go through the motions? Need motivation? Get a training partner. Can't find one? Put an ad in the paper. Do you do the basic exercises or make excuses why you can't? Do you bring each set other than warmups to complete muscular failure where another repetition would be absolutely impossible? If you had a gun put to your head, could you do one more rep?

What is a Champion?

I'm tired of former drug addicts and criminals who are glorified because they have changed and are rehabilitated. The real heroes and champions of life are the ones who never did the drugs and never got in trouble. They did the right thing consistently. A champion is not the reformed steroid user either. Real champions would *never* dream of using drugs. Take down the pictures of steroid users from your gym walls and replace them with pictures of the old-timers or anyone that you could bet your life never took drugs. Have no respect for any drug user. If you say that you're against drugs, then you can't give drug users a place of honor and respect in your life.

True champions are committed to maximize their mental, physical and spiritual potential. They do their best to eat right, train hard, get enough rest, do CV training and stretching, and be totally committed to a healthy lifestyle.

Forget the garbage about living the lifestyle of a competitive bodybuilder. Just focus on getting as strong and healthy as you can. Maximize your physical potential! Champions are people who do the best they can day after day after day. They have a philosophy and they don't just believe in it; they live by it.

BOOK REVIEW:
Dinosaur Training by Brooks Kubik

November 1996

If you have not yet ordered Brooks Kubik's new book, *Dinosaur Training: Lost Secrets of Strength and Development*, don't wait any longer: *order it!* This book is destined to be a classic, and all serious Iron Game fanatics must have it in their collection. This is not a rehash of previously written articles. This is all new information, the kind of stuff hardcore guys like to read.

If you want to "tone up," firm, shape, bodysculpt or just get in shape, this book is not for you! If you like spandex, tanning salons, chrome, sweatbands, wrist wraps, lifting gloves, wear cologne to the gym, and think that sweating to the oldies is hard training, this book is not for you! This book does not cater to sissies and has a definite target reader: The tough, old-time, hardcore drug-free type.

Serious hardcore strength training ideas fill every page. The theme is functional in nature, not cosmetic. This book does not talk about getting striations in your deltoids, the words "buns" and "six-pack" are not mentioned, and there is not a mention of mega-hype supplements. This book is about training brutally hard and getting as strong and massive as you possible can, *naturally*, without taking steroids. This book is about maximizing your potential for size and strength.

If you appreciate Iron Game history and admire old-timers, you will love this book. It cleverly combines historical information and the forgotten training philosophies of our Iron Game pioneers with modern training application. I truly believe that for developing strength, some of the old classics had some of the most productive training programs ever written. Brooks has given new life to many of these ideas. Thick-bar training, odd lifts, one-hand lifts, grip work, and odd-object lifting abound. I never dreamed of using a sandbag until about 18 months ago when I was fortunate enough to be one of the reviewers of *Dinosaur Training*. Try to walk around the block with a 200-lb sandbag and you'll have the workout of your life. *Dino Training* is crammed with information you can use!

Even at 192 pages there are no wasted chapters like so many other books where the author has finished long before the book ends, and wastes space and your time talking about stuff like organizing your weight room or the scientific principles of how a lifting belt works. Every page of this book is functional, informative, and motivational.

I've saved motivation for the end of the review because this is probably the most dominant trait of this book. If you are not fired up and ready to train after reading just a few pages of *Dinosaur Training* then you are in need of a checkup from the neck up. This book will have you so excited about training that you may have trouble sleeping after reading it!

This book is worth many times the modest price. Order it today! If you are serious about strength training, and love the Iron Game, there should be no question; it's a "No Brainer." Get this book, get strong and massive, and maximize your potential without drugs! Hail to the Dinosaurs!

To see all of the great products offered by my good friend Brooks, please visit his website at BrooksKubik.com

TRAINING AND EATING IN THE BIG APPLE

November 1996

I arrived at Penn Station in New York City and walked to the corner of 34th and 8th to meet "The Human Wall," (6'4'', 310-lb) Drew Israel. We both had a great time when Drew visited my place, in Washington, D.C. Now it was time for round two.

Just like clockwork, at 11:15 AM, a car came by close to the curb and the door popped open. It was Drew. It was a good thing that the train was not late. I jumped in, and we were off to eat a pre-workout lunch at the Dixie Pig, one of Drew's and Dr. Ken's favorite places to eat. The place is not fancy, and not in one of New York's better neighborhoods, but the food is great and the portions are huge.

After lunch it was off to Drew's apartment/gym. We talked training and watched a few training videos while waiting for our food to digest. I had to sit between two Hammer machines to see Drew's TV which is mounted high on the wall above another machine. Drew has a large training video collection featuring high-intensity workouts and lectures from top strength coaches. We watched "Strength Training by the Experts" and "Dr. Ken at West Point." We were really fired up to train! Since we were planning to visit Dr. Ken at Iron Island Gym tomorrow, I made damn sure we did all of our training today at Drew's.

Drew initially called me a few years ago after an that described my living conditions at the time. I had literally lived in a gym for several years. Drew didn't think there was another guy as crazy as he was. We had an immediate bonding and have been good friends since. I have since moved my gym into a commercial space, but Drew is still living in his gym.

Drew's gym is an awesome display of dedication and passion for training and the Iron Game. It is a basement studio apartment in a nice Queens neighborhood. He has a bed in the corner, and a bathroom, which are the only two places where equipment is not taking up the entire space. (Later that night I slept on the floor between the Hammer Iso-Lateral Leg Press and Pullover machines. I felt right at home!) Drew has more machines and equipment than some large commercial gyms have. The machines and equipment are packed side by side, many actually touching each other. You have to contort your body just to move around the room.

The Training

We were now ready to train and this time I went first. Drew had me start with the Hammer Chest Press and, after warmups, I did sets of 325 for 8 reps, and 370 for 5 reps. I felt strong and was going to try 400. I took about two minutes rest as this would be a personal record for me, and I wanted it. Drew was yelling encouragement but his shouts faded into the background as my concentration grew intense. I felt good. This was it! *Bam!* It went up about three quarters of the way. I hit a slight sticking point but kept pushing. I rammed it through to lockout. A new PR! No matter what happened during the rest of the workout, I would be happy about this one.

The next movement was on the Tru-Squat® machine from Southern Exercise. I have heard good things about this machine but had never actually had a workout on one. Let me tell you that it was *brutal*. This is a fine piece of equipment that makes you squat with perfect form. It takes all the stress off your lower back and is *harder* than free-weight squats. I will get one of these machines in the future. After warmups I did 20 reps with only 200 lbs and it was *murder!* The poundages on this machine do not correlate with free-weight squats as I've done 380 x 20 in the barbell squat. The 200 x 20 on the Tru-Squat was harder! After completing the twentieth rep I felt sick and had to rest a few minutes.

47

I felt okay after a few minutes and went over to the Hammer Pullover machine. I did a couple of high-rep sets to failure and then weaved my way outside to Drew's driveway where he does his free-weight exercises. There is no room for free weights inside his apartment. Drew has a garage with a bench for bench presses, a lot of free weights, Trap Bar, and other equipment. Trap bar deadlifts, military presses, bench presses, etc., are done in the driveway, even in January! Seated military presses were next in my workout. After warmups I did a set of 8 reps with 190 lbs, and then 210 for 5 reps. I quickly moved back inside Drew's apartment to the Hammer Pulldown and did a few high-rep sets to failure with 180. Workout over! I was still feeling the effects of the Tru-Squat machine.

Now it was Drew's turn to battle the iron. Drew's first exercise was the Hammer Iso-Lateral Leg Press and, after warming up, he did 3 sets of 10 with 550! He lowered the weight slowly and did not bounce at all. An awesome display of strength. After a short rest it was over to the Hammer Chest Press. After warmups Drew did a set of 10 with 380 lbs. When Drew goes all-out to failure he really is at true failure. He looks like he is having a seizure on his last rep!

Drew quickly moved over to the Hammer Pullover machine, his favorite upper-body movement. After warmups he did a gut-busting set to failure with 250 lbs for 15 reps. Drew scraped and contorted himself through the machines and made it to his driveway for seated military presses. After warming up he took 235 lbs for 6 reps, then collapsed. He laid on the grass near the edge of his driveway for a few minutes, before getting up. I was feeling a lot better by now, but we waited a little while for Drew to regain his senses. You can tell when Drew is feeling good because he talks about eating. After about ten minutes Drew began ranting about Peter Luger's Steakhouse ("Petah Loogiz" in New York dialect).

The Eating

I was really looking forward to visiting what Drew calls "the best steakhouse in the world," in the Williamsburg area of Brooklyn. This is an area where you would not walk alone after 5 PM. It is a famous place, known for its huge portions of beef and has been an institution since 1887. It is also one of Dr. Ken's (and the Iron Island gang's) favorite places to eat. Two of Drew's training partners, 6' 260-lb Jim Duggan, and 6'3'' 260-lb Howard Menkes, were going with us. Jim is well known in the New York area but is one of the best kept secrets in the Iron Game. He is one of the strongest drug-free guys in the world. Howard is a strong man in his own right and a big advocate of hip-belt training. He has got great results with it after a back injury. We were soon on our way. The car had tough springs as it carried about 1,000 lbs.

When we got to Peter Luger's we were seated but were rubbing shoulder to shoulder. We had to pull the table a few feet from the wall, which caused a stir. We had to sit straddling the legs of the table so we would have room to move and breathe. There is no menu. It is simply steak for one, two, three, etc. We each ordered steak for two. The four double platters covered the table and there was little room for the bread and side orders. Everyone was staring at us and seemed to be wondering, "Who are those guys?" The steak was great and really hit the spot, especially after a good workout. Drew finished off two baskets of bread, a few side orders, and dessert. I learned a lesson from our last meeting: Do not try to match Drew with a fork or you will regret it! As we were leaving, the manager came over to us and said, "It's been a long time since four guys have come in here and all finished their double steaks!"

After we got back to Drew's place we were both looking forward to a good night's sleep. I crawled between the leg press and pullover machines, and slept like a rock.

Iron Island Gym

The next morning we got up late and all Drew talked about was having lunch at La Palma, a good Italian place. We had a great lunch there and Drew put on a show consuming enough veal parmesan for three people. We then set off on our way to "The Mecca," Iron Island Gym.

When we first got there, I thought it looked small from the front view, due to the store front entrance. Once I walked inside, however, I saw how the place spread out behind the entire row of stores and went back about a block. The place is huge!

When I first walked in, I genuflected. I felt that I was in a sacred place, a place where many great battles have been fought with the Iron. The place was buzzing with enthusiasm and there were people training hard everywhere I looked. It is a hardcore but friendly place, not at all like the typical bodybuilding gym. The walls are covered with pictures and Iron Game memorabilia. It has every type of machine you could imagine, a large powerlifting area, and a graveled area behind the gym where large wheelbarrows and wagons are filled with Olympic plates. You are harnessed to them, and pull them like a mule over the bumpy sand and gravel surface. There are many other unique items there like the lead-filled torpedo cases with welded handles, to use for the farmer's walk, the cannon balls, two custom-made 90-lb Trap Bars, dumbbells with 2 1/2-lb jumps all the way to 200 lbs, and many other unique items.

Dr. Ken has his own custom-made 45-lb plates that are a light purple color (Iron Island Purple) and have IRON ISLAND in white letters that go around the inside of the plates. Drew brought a few of these plates down to my place during his visit. One thing that you will notice right away about Iron Island Gym is that it is extremely neat, with every item in its proper place. There are no plates laying on the floor, and plates are not even left on the equipment after use. Ken has his members trained to put all plates back on the plate racks after they finish their last set on any exercise. They all do it.

Meeting Dr. Ken was great. I spent some time with him in his office and we talked training. I had a great time. I picked up a good training tip that I've applied to my program. It's the fifties day. Dr. Ken has written about this, and Drew uses it in his program. It is not a way to train all the time, but for a change of pace, once or twice a month. I have a new tradition at Whelan Strength Training where everyone's first workout of every new month is fifties day. I pick four or five of the most demanding exercises and the workout's objective is to get 50 reps in each exercise. I do it slightly different than Ken and Drew. I load the bar (or machine) to a weight only slightly lighter than what would normally be used for a set of 10 reps. The client then has to go to failure several times to get to 50 reps. I usually have them do two exercises back to back. They must keep going back and forth until 50 reps of each exercise are done. It is brutal! And it is especially brutal if the exercise selections are the squat (or Trap bar deadlift), bench press, Hammer Iso-Lateral Leg Press, and Hammer Pulldown.

Another good tip I picked up from Dr. Ken is the use of the half-hour workout. I now offer both half-hour and full-hour workouts to my clients. This past year I've added five Hammer Strength units to my gym and this makes life a lot easier and faster. I can "clock" someone in 30 minutes or less now because changing plates is a breeze. When I had only free weights I'd spend at least 15 minutes in any workout changing plates and moving bars and benches around, and in and out of the power rack, etc. Also, a lot of good, tough, young (but broke) guys wanted to sign up with me but couldn't afford the hourly rate. They can now train with me using the half-hour workout option. The shorter workout is just as tough as the hour one, and perhaps even tougher because get little if any rest between sets.

I had a great time in New York, and Iron Island Gym is a must-visit place for all Iron Game fanatics. But soon it was time to head to the train station and catch the train back to Washington. After saying farewell to Ken and Drew I told them I'd be back for another visit, when I attend the Oldetime Barbell and Strongmen Association meeting in October. Then we will have Peter Luger's Round Two. I can't wait!

DINOSAUR WOMEN

January 1997

It was a steamy early-September Saturday in Washington, D.C., and it would be hard *not* to break a sweat. I glanced at the day's schedule and noticed that I had a great lineup of hard workers coming in, and most of them were women! Overall, about one third of my clients are women and they all train *hard*. They are tough and not looking for any mercy. (And they don't get any.) They hate *toning*; they want to get *strong*. They are tired of being underestimated. They want to kick ass and take names! I train them the same as the guys, and they love it. As Charlene McNamara puts it, "Women are tired of being babied!"

I was fired up and really looking forward to getting "in the trenches." I eagerly prepared for the day's coming battles. I filled all the water bottles and put them in the fridge, turned on all the fans, and then got the day's training logs ready. I put a US Marine Corps cadence tape in the stereo and upped the volume. We were ready for *war*, with women at the front lines!

All-out Effort!

First in would be Andrea Rippe. Andrea is 27 years old, 5'3'' and about 134 lbs. She is tough, hard working, motivated and is stronger than most men her size. She is hardcore and wouldn't be caught dead wearing lifting gloves! I put her on the Stairmaster for five minutes to elevate her core body temperature, and then had her do a few minutes of 20-second static-hold stretches. While she was doing this, I pre-loaded all the bars and Hammer machines so we could blast through the workout with minimum delay.

We started things off with the bench press. After warmups we progressively added weight for the first two sets, done to failure, and Andrea completed her last set of 3'' monster-bar bench presses, going to failure on the eighth rep with 130 lbs.

Next was the Hammer Iso-Lateral Row with custom-made 2''
handles. Andrea put some chalk on her hands and then went
through a killer breakdown set of 110, 90 and 70 all done to high-
rep failure. She only got enough rest for me to strip off the plates
and it was *go again.* Her rear delts, forearms and lats were
"cooked."

Next was the deadlift with my Sutherland giant 100-lb Trap Bar
with thick handles. After warmups, it was loaded to 175 lbs and
Andrea took it to failure doing 19 reps. She had to lean against the
Hammer Iso-Lateral Behind Neck Press machine to stay on her
feet, and was breathing so hard that she could probably be heard on
the next floor!

Next was the Hammer Pulldown for 3 sets of 10 with 80 lbs, and
then it was over to the Hammer Iso-Lateral Behind Neck Press
with a breakdown set of 80, 60 and 40, with each set going all out
to failure. Her shoulders were smoking! I had her get right up for
some manual resistance shoulder work, which made her scream.
The place sounded more like a slaughter house than a gym! I let
her take a minute's rest to drink some water.

The next movement was standing reverse curls with a 2''-diameter
bar, and Andrea did 3 sets of 10 reps with 50 lbs. Then it was over
to the Hammer Iso-Lateral Leg Press. She pounded out 2 sets of 20
with 190 lbs with a dead stop pause on every rep. No bouncing
allowed! After the last set of leg presses she was very wobbly. I let
her take a two-minute rest so she could complete the workout. The
"main meal" was over and now it was time for "dessert."

I grabbed the 2''-diameter wrist roller that has a 15'-long rope, and
we headed to the stairway banister. There is no air conditioning in
the stairway and where Andrea was standing was like a sauna!

After a few 15' reps she was "fried" and drenched in sweat. Her
forearms and 14'' arms were swollen and gorged with blood. She
was breathing like a freight train and struggling to suck in enough

air to stay on her feet. She was determined to finish strong and not be KOed. She was soon ready to accept today's final challenge.

At a bodyweight of only 134 lbs she was about to do battle with the 175-lb sandbag, to put the finish on a brutal one-hour high-intensity workout. If she got it, she would be the first woman to transport 175 lbs of sand all the way around the tough course.

Andrea loves the sandbag carry exercise and even has her own sandbag at her house that she practices with. (She is also one of several clients that I've had call Brooks Kubik to jokingly "cuss him out" for introducing me to this torturous device!) She is currently one of only two women with her name already on the 150-lb bag, Charlene McNamara being the other. They have a friendly rivalry that motivates each of them to work even harder.

Women can get their names on the sandbag, and a free workout, if they can carry 150 lbs around the course in under ten minutes. They are not allowed to drag the bag or to put it on their shoulders. It must be "carried" in bear-hug fashion.

My clients frequently make bets with each other, usually offering to pay for a workout, to see who is first to get a certain poundage around the course in less than the ten-minute time limit. The time limit can make things interesting indeed!

A few months ago Charlene McNamara made a (workout) bet with Vern Veldekens that she would get 150 around in under ten minutes before Vern could get 225 around. Since clients can train on different days, the rule is that they have to match the bet on their very next workout to tie, or else they lose. Vern took the bet and, unexpectedly, Charlene got 150 all the way around the very next week. She immediately called Vern and really enjoyed giving him the news.

Vern had just got back from a month-long end-of-semester vacation, and was slightly out of shape. Since he had to do the sandbag carry at his very next workout, he looked doomed to lose this bet. But Vern was determined not to let Charlene beat him, and managed to get the 225-lb bag three quarters of the way around the course in quick time. But this great effort took its toll and when Vern collapsed, he could not even think of getting up for 7 minutes!

I warned Vern of the time and he struggled to get up. He was operating on auto pilot and willed himself to get the bag to within 10' of the finish line, before collapsing again. This time he was almost in a coma.

As the clock ticked away, it looked hopeless. I screamed, "Ten seconds, Vern. C'mon—finish it!" Somehow, Vern jumped up, grabbed the bag, took three big steps and then *dove* across the finishing line, bear-hugging the bag which landed on top of him as the clock ticked to zero! It was a tie and no one won the bet.

Vern stayed down on the floor for a long time and was breathing so hard that it sounded like a tornado, but he had a smile on his face. The first thing he did when he got up, twenty minutes later, was call Charlene.

I let Andrea rest for about three minutes to regain her strength and get her mind ready for combat. "C'mon Andrea, you made 150 look easy. Be the first woman to get 175. Let's do it!"

Andrea attacked the bag and wrestled with it to get it into the clean position. She couldn't quite lock her fingers around the bag, lost her balance and fell over backwards. She was okay, and we had a good laugh. Then she tried it again. Her whole body shook as she struggled to get the bag above her knees. She gave a great heave and screamed with concentrated anger at the bag! She finally had it where she wanted it, in a bear-hug position. This time, she managed to lock her fingers and began her walk around the third floor. She collapsed twice, each time requiring several minutes of rest to regain her sense. She managed to carry the bag more than three quarters of the way around the floor as the ten-minute time limit expired. This was a great workout and a tremendous effort.

Andrea will soon get 175. It's only a matter of time.

Muscle Fiber is Human

Charlene McNamara was next and she went through the same brutal one-hour workout that Andrea did, and ended up also trying to get the 175-lb bag around. She managed to get it about half of the way around, which was quite impressive since she almost killed herself when she got the 150.

Charlene is a *hard* worker and very competitive. The quickest way to get Charlene to do something is to tell her that she can't. She is one of the most determined people I've met. She loves grip work and has an extremely strong handshake. She loves to crush men's hands and make their eyeballs pop out! Ask Mike Thompson and Drew Israel about her vice handshake, as they both have met Charlene.

Stephanie Jirard and Rochelle Bratton are hot on the trail of Andrea and Charlene. They train extremely hard. In fact, most men have probably never trained as hard as any of them. It's by word of mouth, but every week I get a new hardcore dinosaur woman come in who wants to train *hard*. It's great!

Muscle tissue is not defined as male or female, but as *human*. The same principles of intensity and progression apply to training women as they do to training men. Women do not want to be babied! Women should not be embarrassed or afraid to develop strength or to maximize their physical potential. Toning is nothing more than low standards and surrendering to the norms of society.

Toning is an inferior way to train with weights, and a growing number of women want nothing to do with it!

BALANCED TRAINING ROUTINES

March 1997

A few weeks ago, I had a trainee named Tom come by for a consultation and workout. Tom has been lifting for about seven years, is 25 years old 5-8 tall and about 180 lbs. Tom stated that his best bench press (with a regular-diameter bar) was about 302 lbs, but his squat was not much more than that.

We went through our first workout and Tom worked real hard, but I noticed that he had a severe strength imbalance between his upper and lower body. His upper-body pushing and pulling strength was also "out of whack." He could get 8 reps in the bench press with 215 lbs using a 3-inch diameter bar, but had a hard time handling 140 in the Hammer Iso-Lateral Row. He could get 150 for 8 reps in the military press but could not chin himself more than 3 times. To balance his strength and development, Tom needed to put more emphasis on his lower body, and on his upper-body pulling movements.

It was obvious that Tom had spent a great deal of his training time on his back doing bench presses. He had good development of his chest and front delts, but had far less development in his legs, hips, rear delts, and upper back. It was all a matter of thinking. Tom never put an emphasis on working his legs or upper-body pulling movements. As long as his bench press and military press were going up, Tom was happy. (He always did his curls, too.) Tom's ego was not attached to working legs or upper-body pulling like it was to upper-body pushing exercises. Pulling exercises had second class status in Tom's mind, and he would just go through the motions with them and get them in when he could. After our session Tom realized that for the last seven years he had been consistently training only about half of his muscles. He demonstrated that he could train hard when he put his mind to it, but he needed to change his thinking and apply himself to his *entire* body.

Program Design

When designing training programs, always start with the major lower-body work. This separates the men from the boys. Nothing puts the spotlight on a phony quicker (and makes me laugh harder) than someone with a big upper body and an undeveloped lower body. They are in every gym.

Whenever I meet someone who claims to train hard, I can usually tell by their lower-body development if they are telling the truth. Major lower-body exercises, i.e., the squat, deadlift and leg press, are the most demanding of all exercises. Anyone who does not put a primary importance on them gets no respect from me. Squats, leg presses and deadlifts are the top priority and should set the foundation for your balanced training program. Once this is done, *then* you can get the upper-body pushing and pulling in balance.

Some advocates of abbreviated training are designing training programs that are not balanced. Of course it is better to do "less" than "too much," but it is *even better* to do the *right amount* of exercise using a balanced program. Most coaches, myself included, put a high value on the three big basic exercises—squat, deadlift and bench press. The problem, is that many people overlook several other equally important exercises. Their program design usually has a poor balance between pushing and pulling—usually not enough pulling. I have read many articles where the authors have gone to great lengths to describe in detail the upper-body pushing part of a program, and then they add something like, "Throw in a rowing motion to round out the program." That, for many, takes care of the pulling part of a training program.

Some exercises, such as the bench press, are directly connected to the ego of many individuals. This is okay so long as you don't get carried away. The bench press is an important exercise, but it is *no more important* than the Hammer Iso-Lateral Row (or your horizontal pulling movement of choice). Pulldowns or chins are no less important than overhead presses. Don't get hung up on any one particular exercise. You should strive for balanced strength and muscular development. But I am not advocating the de-emphasis of the bench press or any other *major* movement—they are all equally important.

I recently had a phone conversation about this subject with my friend, Dan Riley, the Strength and Conditioning Coach of the Washington Redskins, and one of the most respected people in the field. Dan is a strong advocate of balanced pushing and pulling. My pushing and pulling philosophy is similar to Dan's except that he has more planes of movement due to a much larger facility and access to many more machines. I use the following simple guideline for a balanced upper-body program: a horizontal push, a horizontal pull, a vertical push, and a vertical pull. For the lower body I recently began to rotate the squat, Trap Bar deadlift, and Hammer Leg Press so that each of them is trained once during a period of about ten days, i.e., one of the exercises is trained every three or four days. But some people should deadlift only twice per month because they need a long recovery period for the spinal erectors.

Keep in mind that this is only a helpful checklist that I use. There are some exercises that are not easily put into one of the categories I've just specified, e.g., the pullover and the parallel bar dip. For movements like these, use common sense and define them as either pushing or pulling movements. Then use them as substitutes for other comparable exercises, not as additions to your program.

For many hard gainers, especially those who use multiple work sets of each exercise, there is a serious risk of overtraining if there is too much training volume. You could alternate the vertical and horizontal push and pull and do them once per week each. For example, perform a horizontal push and pull on Monday, and a vertical push and pull on Thursday.

There are many exercises you can use to fill the bill, so you should not go stale. For the vertical push you could use the barbell overhead press, Hammer Behind-Neck Press (which is more like a dumbbell press than a barbell behind-neck press), dumbbell press, or manual resistance. For the vertical pull you could use the chin, pulldown, or Hammer Pulldown. For the horizontal push you could use the bench press, incline press, dumbbell bench press, or Hammer Chest Press. For the horizontal pull you could use the seated cable row, Hammer Iso-Lateral row, dumbbell row while braced against a bench, or virtually any type of machine row that is safe for your lower back.

A balance between pushing and pulling is also important for preventing injuries. Many injuries are caused by muscular imbalance. There is a strong relationship between a joint injury and the development of the musculature that surrounds that joint. Just like a car that pulls to one side when it is out of alignment, your muscles will pull a joint to one side if one side overpowers another. this is at the root of many shoulder, knee and other joint problems.

When designing your training program, always start with the core foundation of your lower body, then move on to balancing your upper-body pushing and pulling. Your body will thank you for it.

SETS FROM HELL!

May 1997

"The mind is its own place and in itself can make
a heaven of hell or a hell of heaven."
—Milton

Big Billy Banks arrived a few minutes early for his Saturday afternoon training session. Even before he got to the door he could hear weights banging, my shouting, and Victor Peck screaming bloody murder through the noisy Marine cadence tape that was blasting away. Billy knew that he, too, was in for one hell of a day!

I have been training Victor (on and off) for seven years. His mother hired me as a present to him for his 30th birthday. He was about 40 lbs overweight at the time, and smoked cigarettes. He had trained a decade earlier but was hobbled by a serious knee injury while playing football, and then he got off track.

Victor is one of the most gung-ho determined guys I know. All he needed was some direction and a little shove. He quit smoking and has taken to serious training like a fish to water. He is now a high-intensity training fanatic and has totally changed his life. He is 6-4 tall and 250 lbs, and in the best shape of his life, at age 37. He has a high level of conditioning and mental toughness, and was an ideal candidate for my new half-hour training program. A bonus is that the half-hour program is much cheaper than the hour-long program. But many people are unable to do the half-hour program because they do not have the high-level of mental toughness that is required. Even many who think that they are in good condition could not take the half-hour workout because every work set is to complete failure with very little rest between sets. *Anyone's* mental (and physical) toughness would be put to the test by the half-hour workout.

I recently twisted Victor's arm to try it. At first he had some doubts. He was used to the hour workout and thought that only half an hour of training wasn't long enough. But now he has no doubts. He is a believer!

Billy joined in with me, screaming at Victor to finish strong. Victor was coming down the home stretch and needed to rally his remaining energy. Victor moved from the Hammer Iso-Lateral Behind Neck Press to the Hammer Iso-Lateral Pulldown—where he went to failure, and then continued to pull in a "static" contraction for an additional 10 seconds. Then it was over to the Hammer Iso-Lateral Leg Press with 350lbs, and Victor pushed out 20 reps. He collapsed in the machine and was drenched in sweat. Prior to Victor's workout the rubber floor was dry. Now there were many small puddles of sweat on the floor.

"Great workout, Bob!" Victor gasped.

"Twenty-seven minutes," I responded, "you worked real hard, as usual."

I asked Billy if he minded starting his workout about ten minutes late, so Victor could do the sandbag. A big grin came over Billy's face. He did not mind at all. Victor wasn't smiling, but he was willing. People love to watch *others* do the sandbag! Victor already has his name on the bag as he got 200 lbs around a few months ago, but had not done it since. He recently tried 225 lbs for the first time, but failed to get it more than 20 feet. Because he was pretty tired, today he was going to go for the 200 again.

For *this* high-rep 30-minute workout we only do warmup work for the first upper-body movement, and the first lower-body movement. The reps are high enough (usually over 10 for the first set of each exercise) for warmup work not to be needed for every exercise. But this system only works if the first set has high reps. If low reps, pyramids or singles were to be used, that would be different and we would do specific warmup sets for *each* exercise (and not be able to fit the workout into a 30-minute session). But Victor was using a very specific routine tailored to fit a 30-minute time limit.

Here is a typical workout that I'll put Victor through in 30 minutes:

Five-minute cardiovascular warmup and series of 20-second static-hold stretches for the entire body.

1. Squat or deadlift (alternating, once per week for each): 1 warmup set and 1 set to failure, moving up in weight next time if 20 reps are reached in perfect form.

2. Hammer Iso-Lateral Chest Press: 1 warmup set, 2 sets to failure.

3. Hammer Iso-Lateral Row: 2 sets to failure.

4. Hammer Iso-Lateral Behind Neck Press: 2 sets to failure.

5. Hammer Iso-Lateral Pulldown: 2 sets to failure.

6. Hammer Iso-Lateral Leg Press: 1 set to failure, moving up in weight next time if 20 reps are reached in perfect form.

Exercises 2-5 are done one after the other, to failure, in two rotating series. The poundage is increased the following workout once 8 or more reps is reached on the second set of a given exercise. Note that exercises 2-5 are alternating pushing and pulling movements. This entire program is done in under 30 minutes, with the hardest exercises done first and last. A sandbag carry and/or grip work is/are sometimes added after the regular 30-minute workout.

Like all of my clients, Victor does cardiovascular work, abdominal work, and extra stretching in his own time.

Sandbag Alley

I recently moved my gym (again) to a bigger and better facility, just a block away from the old place. We now do the sandbag carry outside in a fenced-off alleyway behind the gym. My landlord owns the alley and gave it to me as part of the lease. We call it "sandbag alley." We start and finish at the same place. The actual carry for a single up-and-down trip is about 250 feet. Up and down sandbag alley twice is about the same distance as around the old third floor, so the same 10-minute time limit remains. Victor managed to get the 200-lb bag up and down the alley twice in under 10 minutes before collapsing in a heap. Billy and I were hoarse from screaming encouragement. Victor's workout, including the sandbag carry, took only 35 minutes.

You Can't Train Hard and Long

You can train hard, or you can train long. But you can't do both. One hour is probably the limit for a high-intensity workout. The two- and three-hour marathon workouts in the mega-hype drug-infested bodybuilding mags are greatly exaggerated. Being in a gym for three hours is not the same thing as training hard for three hours. Those guys spend more time looking in the mirror, gossiping and talking than they do training. The drugs they use enable them to train at a low level of intensity and yet still get good results. But most of those types don't have a clue of what a hard workout is.

With my one-hour program (seven exercises) only the third (final) set of each exercise is always done to complete muscular failure, and you get some rest between sets—usually no more than one minute and only after squats, deadlifts and leg presses. For the hour-long workout I use the "controlled failure" method for the first two work sets of each exercise. Using this method you stop at the rep goal for the set, if it's reached. If the goal isn't reached, and you went all out, then you reached muscular failure. The half-hour program (six exercises) has a maximum of only two work sets per exercise, but both are done to complete muscular failure with very little (or no) rest between sets.

Both workouts are brutal and take some getting used to, but I make all newcomers start with the one-hour program. If they adapt well to the program and show that they have the ability to train hard, and are mentally tough, they have the option of switching to the half-hour program.

Here's how Drew Israel describes the difference between my half-hour and one-hour programs: "Bob's hour program is like taking body blows and shots to the head. But the half-hour program is all shots to the head. With both programs you end up on the floor."

My clients have to prove that they are really ready if they want to switch to the half-hour workout. It's not the physical factor I'm looking at; it's mainly the mental factor. To make the half-hour workout productive you must be willing to go all out and hold nothing back. You must be willing "to go down with the ship." You have to have the right mental state to make it work. Many do not. But it's a good system because you get rewarded with a cheaper rate for your mental and physical toughness.

The equipment you have available is a big factor in determining which program would work best for you. You need to have all equipment pre-loaded before starting the workout. If, for example, you only have a single barbell that you use for all exercises, the half-hour workout isn't practical.

Mental Focus

The better your mental focus, the more you are able to get good results from one or two sets to failure per exercise. (To help you increase your mental focus, and effort level, apply what you learn from the excellent article titled "The White Moment," by John

Christy, in *Hargainer* issue #40.) There are many trainees who will not get good results from one or two sets to failure. But it's not because one or two sets to failure doesn't work. It's because the individual has failed to understand and apply what true muscular failure is.

I've been experimenting in my own training with just one set to failure. I've always known that it works, but have never used it. I've always felt better doing at least two sets to failure per exercise. My friendship with Drew Israel influenced me to give it a try. When you see how big and strong Drew is, you can't help but be influenced. Since November 1996 I've only done one set to failure per exercise in my own training. I'm stronger than ever and training with weights for less than one hour per week—two training days per week, less than half an hour for each session. In a recent visit to Drew's place I got 500 lbs for 10 reps in the Hammer Leg Press with a dead stop pause on each rep. (It was the first time I ever used this machine.) It works for me, Drew, and others, because we understand what complete muscular failure is, and what type of mental focus is needed.

Of course, it's important *always* to have good mental focus, but the fewer sets that you do (per exercise), the more important that mental focus is. If you do one set to failure, you can't have a lapse in concentration because you can't make it up in later sets. You must be "on" throughout each set. There is no room for mistakes. Every one must be a quality, all-out kick-ass, life-and-death set or else you will be wasting your time and doing nothing more than burning calories. It's not merely thinking positively. You must combine anger and aggression with positive thinking. *Get mad* at the weights. Growl, scream, and let yourself go! It's life and death. It's combat. You must have the attitude that you are *going to war.* If you can't (or won't) do this, you are better off with multiple sets.

Total Muscular Failure

If you can finish the repetition, then you can't be at positive muscular failure because the weight is still moving in a positive direction. You must try one more rep. Positive muscular failure is not when the weight feels heavy. It's not when you are shaking and your muscles ache. Positive muscular failure is when the weight ceases to move in a positive direction even though you are pushing or pulling as hard as you can. But this is just the first part of a complete set to failure.

The second part of a quality set to true complete failure is continuing to push or pull in a static contraction for about ten seconds after you have reached positive failure. The third and final part of taking a set to complete failure is lowering the weight slowly.

Many exercise scientists and researchers believe that the static contraction (held after reaching positive failure) is the most beneficial part of the set. Whether or not you do it could make the difference between success and failure while using one set to failure. But most people are not willing to train to complete failure because it's so brutal. So one set to failure won't work for these types. These people are not willing to do what it takes to take one set to failure work, but the rewards are great for those who will.

Authors Update: One set to failure is the most TIME EFFICIENT way to train, but you do not need to train to failure to get great results. It all depends on YOU GOAL. As long as you lift heavy and progressive you will get great results. If you do one set to failure with light weight, it is no better than body weight exercise and ceases to be strength training.

FORGET LABELS—JUST TRAIN HARD!

July 1997

Many people make strength training a lot more complicated than it really is. I get phone calls all the time from people who say they want advice but just end up sucking the energy out of me because they can't grasp the simplicity of training. They don't realize that regardless of what mode or method you use, the foundation remains the same.

Many people are looking for a magic formula of success, not advice. They panic when they can't get the *exact* number of reps in the bench press that the training cycle they are following says they should (cycles are a rough guide, but no guarantee of training success). They get hung up on minor details and want to "label" the type of training that I do, or think is "the best." They don't realize that there are many ways to train hard and productively. You don't have to train using just one of them.

Strength training is at least as much art as it is science. Only you know what works best for you. Keep good training notes. Log every workout in detail. Learn from your training. Keep your training simple, because strength training is simple. Don't let academic types confuse you (many of them enjoy doing this). Remember the foundation—train the whole body hard with an equal emphasis on pushing and pulling, with progression as the top priority. Many modes and methods can be used to do this. Focus on the basic multi-joint movements, eat right, and get plenty of rest. That's it! Shake the dust off of your copy of *Brawn*, and reread the book. "Natural," … "Hard,"… "Safe" and "Progressive" are the only labels that are needed to describe your training.

Mix It Up

Even though you should train brutally hard, you should enjoy it! Stuart described this well in *Brawn* as "the joy of effort." It's all a matter of thinking. If you learn to enjoy training hard, you are more likely to be consistent. You will not stick with something that is viewed as drudgery. Enjoy training! One of the best ways to enjoy training is to "mix things up." This will renew the enthusiasm of both your mind and body, as well as produce more balanced conditioning.

I have spent a good deal of my training time doing low reps and singles, but I also do 20-rep squats, 50s days, and high reps. I've used multiple sets for many years but am currently getting good results using only one set to failure for each exercise. I've used both free weights and machines, and have even experimented with various speeds of motion. The point is that many modes and methods work, but it's how you use them that counts. Don't waste energy arguing about which one is "best" because there is no point. Try the different modes and methods yourself.

Every three or four months, change your routine. Make some big changes. Do 20-rep squats for four months, then do 10-rep squats for a while. Four months later, go down to 5 reps. I couldn't imagine doing 20-rep squats all the time! And I couldn't imagine doing low reps all the time either. After about every four months my joints want a change. Train with no rest between sets while doing a brief workout of no more than 30 minutes. Four months later, give yourself some rest between sets and see how heavy you can go! Use your imagination and go with your instincts. Listen to what your body is telling you—only *you* know how you feel. Make the changes needed to keep your enthusiasm high so you can really attack the equipment when you train. Don't get hung up on labels as this only limits the tools you have available for building your body.

I don't train my clients using one rigid training program. I usually start them out with higher reps, and then after several months, when they have a good foundation, we'll try some new things. We do a 50s day once a month (usually the first workout each month), complete with Du-Wop 1950s music blasting on the stereo. (Fifties day means 50 reps each on five different machines, for a one-hour workout.) As my clients come in the door and hear Buddy Holly or the Platters (not the marines) they scream, "Oh no! It's 50s day!!" (This makes torture fun!)

Around the 15th of the month, for a change of pace, I'll put my clients through one workout of extremely slow movements. I'm not an advocate of training this way all of the time, but have nothing against anyone who does, as it works for sure. Every two weeks my clients get hammered with something radically different. It keeps their body shocked and off guard, and morale and motivation high.

For the past two months I've been training Melvin Tuten. Melvin is a huge man, 6-7 and 335 lbs. He is an offensive tackle for the NFL Cincinnati Bengals. Because of the severe flooding in the Cincinnati area, he has stayed home (in Washington, D.C.) during the off-season and has been training with me.

On a recent 50s day Melvin got 540 lbs for 50 on the Hammer Iso-Lateral Leg Press, with a dead stop pause on each rep! He is now doing mainly a moderate to low-rep high-intensity program. But we mix it up and throw in 20 reps on the Tru-Squat sometimes, along with a 50s day, a slow day, sandbag, etc.

Mind Games

Manage your own progression system. I have always believed in progression by performance, not time. All my clients have to earn a poundage increase on the basis of the performance of their previous workouts. I have never believed that you can forecast increases according to a schedule. If you get stuck on a particular poundage, you must learn to be your own sports psychologist and play games with your head.

71

I frequently lie to my clients and don't tell them the weight on the machine or bar, even if they ask. I sometimes tell them that I took off weight when I really added weight. They don't know what to expect, so they can't worry about not getting a certain poundage. As a result they just focus on pushing or pulling as hard as they can.

Anyone who has had success in strength training has had to master their mind. If you train alone, this is more difficult, but this is a challenge you should enjoy and must master if you are to maximize your potential. If, for example, you get stuck with 245 x 5, 5, 4 and can't seem to get the 5, 5, 5 that you want, change the goal for a while. Try a week or two with sets of 4 at 255, try a triple with 265, or a double with 275. Go to failure with 215, or do just 2 sets of 5 and get rid of the third set!

If you keep good notes you can make the proper changes to avoid a mental rut, and have new goals on an almost daily basis. You are your own coach and must find ways to keep your mind positive and fresh. Then go back to 245 after a few weeks, but with a new outlook.

Effort Is The Key

A barbell, Hammer machine, Tru-Squat machine, or dumbbell will not produce good results unless the person using the tool is willing to put forth the consistent effort required. If anyone tries to tell you that they have the "only way to train," or even "the best way to train," don't listen. If they say it is the best way *for them to train*, that's different. But if they use a blanket statement and say they know the best way for everyone to train, they are ignorant. Many times they have something to sell you. They may want you to go along with their "program," buy a book, or pay for a certification program, etc.

Mike Thompson and Drew Israel train very differently if you look at modes and methods. But so what? Both their approaches work. If, however, you look at the basic core foundation, they are similar and sound. Neither is better than the other. Through trial and error, and by listening to their own bodies, both men have found what they enjoy and what works for them. You should do the same.

BE PREPARED TO TRAIN!

September 1997

*"All of us were young, healthy, tough, and had the attitude
that you had better throw everything you've got at us,
because WE CAME TO TRAIN!"*

—Dr. Ken Leistner

There are many people who truly believe they are doing the best they can, but they are holding back. I get them all the time. Sometimes it takes them weeks or even months before they really understand what an all-out set to failure really is, and the total commitment it takes to do it right. Usually it is a casual attitude and a lack of preparation that holds them back. They are either mentally or physically *un*prepared to give an all-out effort. Subconsciously they do things to sabotage their training because deep down they really don't enjoy it.

To get the most out of your training you must *want* to train hard. *No one* can help you if you don't help yourself.

Once you decide that this is what you really want to do, and it is not just the latest fad you are involved with, you must seriously prepare for each workout. Training success is nothing more than a long string of consistent high-quality workouts. You take each "one at a time" while being prepared to make each set as productive as possible.

Mental Preparation

Clear your mind of problems and other concerns before you being training. You need to have all your mental energy focused on battling iron. Talking should be kept to a minimum, and if you do talk, don't jump into your next set without refocusing your mind. Take about 20 seconds to get your mind in gear (tell you friends to shut up!) and totally concentrate on how you will very shortly be going all out. If you don't do this, your mind will be on what you were just talking about, not on training, and you will produce a submaximal effort. Remember, you should *have your mind ready for war* when you train.

I have all my clients order *The Magic of Thinking Big* by David Schwartz, one of the best motivational/positive thinking books ever written. You should do the same. You can order it at any major book chain (or BobWhelan.com). And order *The Psychology of Winning DVD's* by Dennis Waitley.

Warming Up

One of the most neglected and important elements of productive training is a good warmup. Your chance of getting injured is considerably lower if you take the few minutes to warm up. you will also perform better because your muscles will be prepared to go all out.

Before you lift any weights, a cardiovascular warmup (stationary bike, stairclimber, etc.) should be done for 5-10 minutes—to "preheat" your muscles and elevate your core body temperature. But don't go too long as this is just a CV warmup *not a CV workout.* Once you are warm and sweating—after about 5-10 minutes—that's long enough. Going longer is not beneficial and may make you weaker by robbing glycogen from your muscles and liver that should be used for your strength-training workout. This warmup should be followed by a series of static-hold stretches of at least 20 seconds each for the whole body. This should be done before *every* workout.

Metabolic/Cardiovascular Conditioning

Your metabolic conditioning (i.e., your ability to train *hard,* without excessive rest between sets, for the duration of the *entire planned workout* and without getting KOed) is greatly enhanced if you are doing *regular* CV training.

One of my pet peeves is the abundance of wrong information in "muscle magazines" about CV training. Many authors, usually ex-bodybuilders with no formal education in the exercise field, frequently recommend doing CV training only twice per week. They are concerned with cosmetics (their bodyfat level), not training their hearts. Twice per week is not enough, and three times per week is only the *minimum* for cardiovascular exercise. Three to five times per week is the proper range. This is not my opinion but that of The American College of Sports Medicine and almost every respected organization in the fitness field.

USA Today had an article a few years ago which stated that "weekend warriors," or people who do less than the minimum of three times per week of CV training, are at higher risk of "sudden death" in exercise because they never get the desired CV conditioning effect from such a low training volume.

Don't lump exercise into one category, as strength training and CV training are separate and have different rules. Strength training should mainly be considered only as training for your muscles, bones, tendons, ligaments, etc. And CV training should mainly be considered as working your heart muscle and burning fat. Although any exercise is better than nothing for your heart and muscles, in reality your muscles get only minimal strength benefit from CV training; and your heart gets some benefit, but minimal, from strength training. You must do both types of training to be totally fit.

Strength training works the fast twitch fibers and burns only carbohydrates, not fat; CV training works the slow twitch fibers and burns fat predominantly, and, depending on the intensity level, a percentage of carbohydrates. Just because you train with weights twice per week does not mean that you can subtract from the *minimum* for CV training.

Living a long and healthy life is a higher priority than adding 5 lbs to your bench press, *but you can do both!* Remember, your goal is not to look big in your coffin!

Your Muscles Can't Compensate for Poor Fuel

Since you can't use your fat storage for an energy supply during strength training, it is critical that you have a good supply of glycogen stored in your muscles and liver before you work out. You should consume about 300-400 calories of carbohydrate approximately two hours before you train. People who don't train *hard* probably don't need to do this, but if you are doing a high-intensity workout, especially if you train for over 45 minutes, you burn a tremendous number of calories (from carbohydrates).

If you ever have that *weak* feeling during a workout, like you are "out of gas," it is because you have burned all your carbs and are out of fuel. Top off the "tank," like you do with the car before a long trip, and you should not run out. Have some pasta, rice, potatoes, etc., about two hours before you train and you will be breathing steam! But for those who train early in the morning, it's nearly impossible to do this without ruining a good night's sleep. Getting up at 4 AM to eat for a 6 AM workout, for example, would ruin your night's sleep. If you train early in the morning you can drink a carbohydrate drink available at most health food stores. (Everything at health food stores is not garbage, just most things—and I'm only half kidding.)

Getting ALL Your Work Done

Tim Denhoff has been training with me for about four months, and has made good progress. It took him about six weeks, however, before he could train for an hour without feeling sick. We xperimented with every possible exercise sequence, doing legs last, taking long rests between sets, keeping reps for legs in the moderate range, etc. But I always managed to get his whole body worked even if the planned workout was cut short. Your top priority should be to finish the planned workout. It is better to modify your exercise sequence to accomplish this than to stick with a larger-muscles-first (legs) philosophy if you can't then finish your workout.

Most of the people that I like and respect the most, guys like Dr. Ken and other hardcore high-intensity types, usually do their leg work first. This starts off the workout with a *bang!* You are breathing heavily and dripping in sweat right off the bat. This sets the tone for the rest of the workout and is probably the norm for many hardcore guys. This makes the rest of the workout harder and raises the intensity level "big time."

Doing a couple of sets to failure in the squat or Trap Bar deadlift to begin a workout is also good when you want to send a message. For example, I remember a couple of years ago when a guy (who made sure, over the phone, I knew how tough he thought he was) called me about training. I didn't like his overly cocky attitude and, since he was not a beginner, and claimed to have been training hard for years, I thought I'd test him. In his first workout I hammered him right off the bat with high-rep leg work. I had him do 20-rep Trap Bar deadlifts immediately followed by 20 reps in the Hammer Leg Press. That knocked him out, workout *over!* The guy's attitude was permanently changed.

Working legs first is great if you like to do it that way. But it is very tough. Some people, and especially beginners, would be better off doing legs at the end of their planned workouts. I know from experience that people don't like paying for an hour's workout if they train (doing legs first) for only 15 minutes and then spend the next 45 minutes hugging the toilet bowl! Training hard should be everyone's goal, but if you knock yourself out early and don't finish all the planned work, you are selling yourself short. Design your program in a manner that makes you enjoy your training and enables you *to finish all the planned work.*

There are few absolute rules in strength training, and this applies to exercise sequence. Working the largest muscles first is usually a good rule, but I believe a better description of this rule would be to work the largest muscles of *either* the upper body of lower body first (by the use of multi-joint movements), before you do any isolation exercise for the same areas. By using this revised rule you can work upper body first, which for some people is better. If, for example, you are wiped out after deadlifts or squats (or even just impaired) and you do them first, the rest of your workout will suffer. If you get KOed, the workout will be over. My goal as a coach is to get you through the entire workout but have you teetering on the edge the whole time. A work of art would be to have you KOed on the last set of the workout.

Enjoy your training but be prepared both mentally and physically before each workout. Many of the elements of preparation are small details, but they add up to a big difference in the results you achieve.

GETTING PERVIS BACK IN SERVICE

November 1997

I was checking my messages in mid-July and heard, "Hi Bob, this is Shaun Brown, the strength and conditioning coach of the Boston Celtics. I'd like to speak with you about the possibility of training Pervis Ellison, who lives in the DC area in the off season, until he reports to us in Boston in late September." That was a phone call I answered right away! I was born and raised in the Boston area and have been a Celtics fan my whole life. There is no other team in the world that I would rather help.

After I spoke with Shaun he said he would call Pervis to see if he was interested, but Pervis had to be willing. This had to be a voluntary decision, not one forced upon him. If Pervis did not want to do it, that would be the end of it. As it turned out, Pervis was very interested, and willing to try anything to revive his basketball career. Pervis is a 6-10 center, and was the first player chosen in the NBA draft in 1989. He won the NCAA championship while at the University of Louisville, but so far has not reached his full potential in the pro's due to his many injuries.

The Background

While in college, Pervis was nicknamed "Never Nervous Pervis" for his clutch play in playoffs. In the pro's, however, it's been a different story. Danny Ainge, a former teammate of Pervis with the Sacramento Kings, nicknamed him "Out of Service Pervis." Pervis has had both of his knees operated on twice. His left knee, especially, has been giving him problems since he shattered his left knee cap a few years ago. Over the last few years Pervis has spent more time in the whirlpool than on the court. But when he plays, he does great. He has excellent production based on time played.

80

A few days later, Shaun flew down to my place in Washington and we went over Pervis' training. We hit it off well, as our training philosophies are very similar. Shaun is a no-BS hardcore guy. He has to be to work for Rick Pitino, the Celtics' new coach and President, who is a fanatic about team strength and conditioning. (Shaun also worked for Coach Pitino at The University of Kentucky.) The Celtics have gone from "the outhouse" to "the penthouse" as far as their strength and conditioning program is concerned. According to Pervis, last year the players were "on their own" for strength training. They would just "dabble with the weights" when they felt like it. Their equipment was little more than a Universal machine. This year, under Rick Pitino and Shaun Brown, they will have about fifteen new Hammer Strength machines to work with. They will have even more equipment next year when their state-of-the-art training complex is finished. They will also have Shaun Brown "in their faces" for every workout. They will be one of the best, if not the best conditioned team in the league.

Pervis arrived a little later, with his agent Bill Strickland. We all found a machine to sit on (or lean against), as I have no unused space. Shaun did most of the talking, explaining to Pervis our training program. Pervis has never consistently trained hard with weights.

Pervis has been with poor, losing teams his whole pro career—ones that had poorly-run strength-training programs. Shaun and I both believe that what Pervis needed was to train his whole body hard and consistently, with an organized and personalized high-intensity program. His knee problems were mainly cartilage ones (not tendon or ligament) that have been repaired (or "cleaned out") surgically. We were not going to retreat from working his legs. Not working his legs has got him nowhere in the past except to the whirlpool. We were going to attack the problem and have him work his whole body with emphasis on his legs, to strengthen his "weak link" and make his knee joints more stable. Pervis was enthusiastic and ready to get started.

Getting Down to Business

We then put him through a workout, but did not hit him too hard. Shaun and I both took turns to work him, but we did not want to "cripple" him and scare him away. I wanted him to come back. Our next workout was in just a few days and I didn't want any cancellations. Pervis thought he had been put through the wringer during that first workout, but he hadn't seen anything yet.

During Pervis' first workout (in front of his agent) we found out important things about his training, such as prior injuries, range of motion limitations, proper poundage to use, and any pain felt. He had no upper-body problems. Only his knees "sometimes" bothered him. We started each exercise light and moved him up to find the right training poundages to start out at. We also found the correct settings for him in machine exercises.

Once his training poundages and range-of-motion adjustments were documented, he was ready to go for the next workout. (On the Tru-Squat, I started him on a partial squat, down to only about 6 inches above parallel. Then over the course of a few workouts I moved him, hole by hole, down to parallel-depth squatting.) Remember that Pervis is a professional athlete and only 30 years old. Even with his gimpy knees he is in tremendous shape when compared to the average person off the street. A regular middle-age guy off the street would need several weeks as an adjustment/break-in period before training hard.

The next workout I gave Pervis the same two-hour orientation that I give everyone else. I also had him order *The Psychology of Winning* and *The Magic of Thinking Big* (see last issue), and gave him a copy of *Brawn*. After orientation I had Pervis do a "Fifties Day" workout. He got a kick out of the fifties music playing. I had him do fifty reps on the Tru-Squat, Horizontal Tru-Press, Hammer Behind Neck Press, Hammer Iso-Lateral Row, and Hammer Pulldown. (A weight was selected for each exercise that was heavy enough to require several sets to failure in order to complete the 50 reps.) We also did some extremely slow reps just for his left leg (weakest knee) on the Hammer Iso-Lateral Leg Press. We did extra stretching, ab work, and grip work, and I even initiated Pervis with a visit to sandbag alley. I had to help him get the 150-lb bag up to bear-hug position, but once he got his arms around it he managed to get it up and down the course. Pervis really worked his ass off!

I push Pervis real hard, but good form always comes ahead of poundage with me. I make Pervis use flawless form to minimize the chance of injuries.

He told me that those 50 reps on the Tru-Squat got his legs and glutes so sore that he had to use his baby's foam-padded toilet training seat for a few days (even though he could barely fit onto - it). Now that's sore! Pervis loves the Tru-Squat (Southern Xercise 800-348-4907, see my article on page 47 of issue #49). But being 6-10 he could never come close to doing a parallel squat with a barbell.

Training Specifics

Pervis' strength-training workouts had a core structure. We always started with a warmup consisting of five minutes of cardiovascular work immediately followed by ab work and static stretching. Then came five multi-joint major movements: (1) Bench Press /Horizontal Tru-Press, (or Hammer Chest Press), (2) Barbell Row /Hammer Row, (3) Barbell Squat or Tru-Squat (or Hammer Leg Press), (4) Military Press or Hammer Behind Neck Press, (5) Pulldowns. I use a lot of variety as some workouts are done with 3 straight sets per exercise, some in breakdown style, some with one arm or leg at a time (i.e., dumbbell style, as all my machines are iso-lateral—can be used one limb at a time), some are done barbell style (i.e., with both arms or legs working simultaneously). Plus once a month there's a fifties day, and at another workout each month there is a slow day. We do a variety of manual resistance almost every workout (especially for inner and outer thighs, and hamstrings). Time permitting we do additional slow work for his weak leg, plus curls, grip work, and a sandbag carry.

I see most of my regular clients only twice a week, for just strength training. Pervis is almost a part-time job. I spend 2-3 hours per day with him, usually four days a week. I do conditioning (e.g., running drills on a basketball court), plus cardiovascular work and extra stretching with him. We train with weights on Monday and Thursday. On Tuesday and Friday we go to Catholic University (where I was the strength and conditioning coach several years ago, and still have a few contacts) to run on the quarter-mile track, swim in the pool, and do running drills on the basketball court. Sometimes he uses the Stairmaster instead of the swimming. I'm pretty much on my own with the strength-training part of the program, but defer to Shaun and follow his program to the letter for the conditioning part.

Results

Pervis is getting stronger each workout, and has gained almost 20 lbs of muscle over the summer. His playing weight was under 235 lbs last year. He is a few pounds over 250 at the time of this writing. He will get even bigger and stronger because Shaun will work him real hard all season long. So far, his knees are feeling better than ever. The intensive running has caused his back some problems and he had to lay off a few times, but nothing serious. To help counter this problem we do a lot of stretching, and alter the intensity of the running. But he will have to be able to run hard to play for Rick Pitino.

Pervis is so big that a 20-lb gain in bodyweight only had the visual effect of a 10-lb gain on a regular-size guy. I advised him to eat a good breakfast every day. He has three main meals that include 5-9 portions of fruits and vegetables, and at least 8 glasses of water per day. A simple vitamin-mineral pill per day was the only supplement he took. I also had him eat two cans of tuna per day (between meals), one in mid-morning and one in the afternoon. So he had five feedings per day. I also encouraged him to drink a lot of skim milk each day. Natural food is the best protein supplement. The strength training has greatly increased his appetite, so he has no problem eating!

Shaun flies down the DC every 2-3 weeks to watch me put Pervis through his paces. The more Pervis sweats and screams, the bigger the smile on Shaun's face. We have daily progress reports on the phone after each workout. Believe it or not, Pervis really likes the strength-training part of the program and realizes how important this could be to his career.

Pervis has made great short-term gains despite the fact that he has missed more than a few planned workouts (especially the running). But when he trains, he really works very hard. He will come to three workouts in a row, and then not show up. Then he will come back and work extremely hard for another week, and then miss a workout. Mind you, considering how well he has progressed, perhaps he needed the unplanned extra rest days in order to fully recover from each group of intensive workouts. Pervis has the potential to be as big and strong as Karl Malone if he applies totally commitment.

Since Rick Pitino took over, the Celtics have made so many roster changes that only a few players from last year remain on the team. Pervis could be a member of the Miami Heat or some other NBA team by the time this article comes out. But I hope he stays with the Celtics and is able to contribute. High-intensity strength training is just what Pervis needs to get back on the court and reach his full potential. If he stays with the Celtics, Shaun will make him train year round. It could be the piece of the puzzle that was missing for him to play regularly and injury-free.

Lessons to Learn

There are many lessons that regular trainees can learn from Pervis' strength training. Even an elite level guy needs to adapt to a new training program, determine safe ranges of motion, apply correct form, train very hard and briefly, eat every three hours or so, follow a sound diet that includes fruit, vegetables and plenty of water, and focus on progressive poundages in good form. The formula works for Pervis and my other clients, and it will work for you too.

NIGHTMARE ON SEVENTH STREET

January 1998

A few months ago Eric Weinstein and Drew Israel drove all the way down to Washington, D.C., from New York City (and drove back the same day) just so I could put Eric through a workout. Drew wanted me to hammer Eric hard like the workouts we had together at my place last year. Eric wanted it that way, too, and was expecting the type of grueling workout that would make Freddy Krueger proud.

Eric is 33 years old, 5'9'' and a solid 195 lbs. He's the throwback type—tough, motivated, strong and extremely polite. I've gotten to know him, Dr. Ken, Jim Duggan, Jamie LaBelle and other members of the "Iron Island gang" pretty well from my visits to Drew's place, and Drew's several previous visits here. Eric and I have trained together at Drew's a few times, and then gone out to Peter Luger's Steak House after the workout. This is not a regular habit for any of us, just a tradition when we all get together.

Eric has been training with Dr. Ken since he (Eric) was 16; he has also trained with Drew for several years. So it goes without saying that Eric has excellent mental focus, and flawless form. Since I knew Eric was a high-intensity-training veteran, I did not have to use the same caution that I would with a beginner off the street.

Eric wanted me to put him through a workout on my turf, to add to his collection. Some people collect stamps, others collect coins. Eric collects workouts. I knew that Eric was used to being hammered by Dr. Ken, so I didn't want to let Eric down. I was pulling no punches and planned on giving Eric a workout to remember.

87

I had the Marine cadence cassette blasting, and after the cv warmup, static holds for his whole body, and a few warmup sets on the machines to be used. Drew and I were shouting encouragement. Eric was psyched and ready! I had him begin with the Southern Xercise Horizontal Tru-Press with custom (Sutherland) 2.5-inch thick handles. The handles alone weigh 30 lbs. Eric went to failure at 10 reps with 140 lbs, and his chest was in real discomfort. (This machine uses about half the poundage of free-weight bench presses, and is a real ego killer!)

Then it was over to the Hammer Iso-Lateral Row for a set to failure with 200 lbs followed by a few forced reps.

As soon as he got off the Hammer machine I had him go to the 2-inch thick bar for a high-rep set to failure with 75 lbs in the reverse curl, with special emphasis on lowering the bar slowly (at least 5-6 seconds per negative). As soon as he hit failure he put the bar down and gave his hands a shake. Then he picked the bar right back up for a set of regular curls (palms up) to failure, again with emphasis on lowering the bar very slowly. As soon as he put the bar down it was back to the reverse curl for a final all-out set. I then let him take a one-minute rest.

Eric repeated this sequence of Horizontal Tru-Press, Iso-Lateral Row and curls two more times, to failure. On the third (last) time he pushed (in the Tru-Press) and pulled (in the Iso Row) for ten seconds in a static contraction after reaching muscular failure. The reverse curls got his forearms bulging and swollen with blood. His hands, wrists and forearms were so "nuked" that he had a hard time holding onto the handles of the Iso Row on the third series.

As soon as Eric had put down the bar after the third series, it was "Get right up!" on the Hammer Iso-Lateral Leg Press for one set to failure with 430 lbs. Each rep was done with a dead-stop pause at the bottom. The seat was set near the "tightest" position so that

Eric's knees sunk into his chest at the bottom. After 10 reps he was

88

breathing like a steam engine, and paused to take ten deep breaths. He made it to 15 reps and then started to scream on every rep. Drew and I were screaming too! "C'mon Eric, get to 20! One at a time...*puuussshhh...*" Eric made it to 20 reps, and was shaking. A few reps later he started to moan between the screams, as he approached the end of the set. He paused to take about fifteen deep breaths and *kept the set going*, with each rep being an all-out, painful, life-and-death effort. He made it to 30 reps before collapsing in the machine. He then rolled to the floor and stayed there for a few minutes. The set was a great effort! Most people would have stopped at 15 reps.

Most people would have been KOed and done with training right now, but not Eric. I knew he would bounce back. He was used to this type of training from all the brutal stuff Ken and Drew do to him. This was just a regular training day for Eric! After a few minutes of rest, we continued. Eric did a few high-rep sets to failure on the Hammer Behind Neck Press with 160 lbs, then a few sets to failure on the Hammer Pulldown with 170, each with a ten-second static contraction on the last set. I threw in some manual resistance for his shoulders, some grip work, and some calf work.

We then went to the Tru-Squat as we wanted to finish with some "ground-based" training. (My tongue-in-cheek definition of "ground-based training," as coined by Jamie LaBelle, is "ending up on the ground" after a hard set, and has nothing to do with having your feet on the ground.) Eric did a set of 20 reps with 200 lbs, which was even harder than and took *more effort* than the leg press set. After the twentieth rep, Eric was on the ground for about ten minutes.

The Tru-Squat is one of the best ground-based training tools because it trains you "into the ground." (For those not familiar with the Tru-Squat, it is an ego killer because you can use only about half the weight of barbell squats.)

After the long rest, Eric felt better. The main course was over. Now it was time for "dessert."

We went outside to sandbag alley where I store my sandbags. Eric was exhausted, but got a second wind after the needed rest and a big glass of water.

He wrestled with the 200-lb bag and carried it over the course of 225 feet in well under the ten-minute time limit. He only put the bag down a few times, and probably could have done 225 lbs. He had been practicing the sandbag carry with Drew, and wasn't coming all the way down here unless he got his name put on the bag.

Drew has been training with over 300 lbs in the sandbag carry. Rumor has it that Drew will attempt 350 lbs to set a new Whelan Strength Training record at the second annual Capital City NSCA Clinic (see ad after this article). Big Melvin Tuten holds the current record of 325 lbs, which he got in his last workout before reporting to the Cincinnati Bengals in July.

Eric slumped for a few minutes against the fence that borders the alley, to let his racing heart and steam-engine breathing get back to normal levels. He did a great job today and worked extremely hard, but was glad the workout was over. All he wanted now was a good meal and a good bed! I put his name on the bag with a magic marker. We were all hoarse from screaming.

Shortly afterwards we headed for Morton's to watch Drew (6'4'' and 310 lbs) set new world records. Nothing like it after a brutal workout. Good workout, good food, good friends; ah, life is good!

EFFORT AND DEDICATION
MAKE MANY METHODS WORK

March 1998

A few years ago, while attending the annual conference of the National Strength and Conditioning Association in New Orleans, I was having a conversation with a well known Ph.D. "researcher type." We talked for about twenty minutes, and seemed to be getting along great. Out of the blue he asked me, "Do you do power cleans?" When I replied that I did not usually do them now but did them for years when I was younger (but I had nothing against him for doing them), he abruptly stopped talking to me and walked away.

There are many jerks in the training field. They think that they alone have all the answers, and if you don't agree with their particular theory or approach, then you are their enemy. Their whole self esteem is based on having you agree with them.

And there are also many narrow-minded robots who can only think in one direction at a time. They take any variation or difference of opinion as a personal insult.

Every time someone thinks he has all the answers, I can find hundreds of strong men who don't train like the know-it-all says they should, but they are usually a lot bigger and stronger than the "expert."

Many of these know-it-all types love to argue, and like to use "science" as their defense. There is a big problem here because every camp has its own version of science. Each uses its own "pet" researchers who espouse the "party line."

91

I hold a Masters degree in exercise science and can tell you that most professors of exercise science look like they never touched a weight in their lives. They can talk forever about the body's physiological response to strength training, but have no clue on how to use the various modes and methods of training.

Many of the leading scientists and researchers don't agree on the best modes and methods of training. Talk to Ted Lambrinides, Wayne Wescott, Ralph Carpinelli, James Graves or Mike Pollock and you may not get the same "scientific" explanation as you would from Mike Stone or William Kramer. And talk to Ellington Darden and you may get something all together different.

There Are Few Absolute Rules in Strength Training

One of the absolute rules I know of is that progressive poundages (lifting heavier), plus good nutrition and adequate recovery, equals good results. I feel sorry for the beginner who reads the "cat fights" and opposite views each backed by "science" as supposedly the best way to train. The beginner may be so confused that he does not know what to do. One author may have "absolute scientific principles" that "prove" you must train "explosively." Then turn the page and the next author says he has the grip on "science" that you must, for example, train using extremely slow reps.

There is a big difference between giving an opinion of what works for you, and giving information that is defined as scientifically "proven" as the "best" way to train. According to Dr. Wayne Wescott, the only significant factor in a successful strength-training program is to train progressively … in the anaerobic energy system. All other facts are minor compared to this, and provide different results for different people.

The Enjoyment Factor

Most people will get best results doing what they enjoy. You can't argue about what someone else likes to do. If you like to train using slow reps, go for it, but don't tell me that I must do it, too, or that I shouldn't be moving my facial muscles or screaming as I train. If you like to train fast (or explosively), and can do it without getting hurt, then do it. Both ways can work, but neither is the best way.

Climbing mountains can be dangerous, but if you have a passion for climbing them you should be able to. It's the same with lifting rocks and sandbags, and doing power cleans or snatches. If you enjoy doing this sort of training, or have a background in Olympic lifting, then do it. I don't perform the Olympic movements now because I don't enjoy them. My background is in powerlifting.

I also don't believe that power cleans, snatches and jerks work as much muscle as other exercise variations. I would rather do deadlifts, rowing, presses and shrugs.

It takes great skill to power clean right and avoid injury. I would rather teach people lifts that don't require as much learned skill to do them. But I don't hate anyone who likes the power clean. It can still be a fine exercise if you do it right.

The Safety Factor

If you are a coach, you have to judge what is best for your athletes or clients considering their different ages, medical backgrounds and injury history. For some people, lifting rocks or sandbags would be crazy. Everyone I train does not perform the same workout. A young tough athlete will be trained extremely hard. A beginner in his forties will be started very carefully and conservatively. *I don't want any deaths in my gym.*

Speed of Motion vs. Poundage

It's common sense that speed of motion and poundage are directly related, and are like the opposite ends of a see-saw. The faster the speed of motion, the heavier the poundages that can be used. And the slower the speed of motion, the lower the poundage that can be used. Both ways can be productive. But the terminology used in the different camps of training is not the same.

Enthusiasts of slow training would be far more effective at winning over opinions if they talked more about progression and getting stronger, and less about minor details and overcomplicating training. Training is not nearly as complicated as they enjoy making it. It seems to me that most slow-speed enthusiasts are more concerned about the strength curve of the machine that the strength of the person using the machine. They love the word "inroads" but don't talk enough about strength and progression. Regular-speed proponents like to talk about strength, poundage and progression. These factors should still be the focus if you are training slow, and are the unifying factors of all methods.

Strength is defined as the ability to produce force. Many conventional-speed trainers believe that slow-rep training with less resistance (force) is simply taking strength training one step closer to calisthenics. Most people fall on one side or the other when it comes to speed of motion, but I see no problem with using more than one rep speed. But you need to understand the difference between poundage and progression.

Progression, Not the Numbers Game

Using the highest possible poundage (or the highest number) is not always the same thing as progression. Poundage comparisons only have validity when comparing the same mode of training and rep

speed. It's possible to use bigger poundages but without necessarily having progressed, just as it's possible to use reduced poundages and yet still make progress.

Certain machine variations of barbell exercises force a considerable reduction in weight used, e.g., the Tru-Squat reduces squatting poundage by 50%. It's the same thing with speed of motion. You will use a lot less weight going at a slower speed. Poundages are only relative when measured against the same modes, rep speeds and equipment. For example, you may Hammer Leg Press 530 lbs for 8 reps at regular speed (2 seconds concentric, 4 seconds eccentric), but only be able to use 375 lbs for 8 reps at 8/8 speed. You should not let the number 530 make you feel inferior if you if you use an 8/8 speed and the accompanying reduced poundage. The workout with 375 lbs may even be harder and take more effort because it's on an entirely different scale to that used for the 530 lbs. *You can't compare numbers at different rep speeds.* Just focus on *progression* within the speed used.

Many people will not even consider using certain machines, or training at a slower speed, because they will have to train with lighter weights. It's an ego thing or numbers game with them. They focus on numbers and not progression.

Don't be hung up on numbers. Focus on progression—i.e. adding weight (using consistently good form, of course)—in the rep speed and/or on the equipment you are using. *Progression, not purely the highest poundage number, is the top priority and the constant unifying factor regardless of the speed of motion or apparatus used.* Slow-rep cadence training has a bad image in the eyes of many poorly-informed conventional-speed people. This is because many people who are not strong are attracted to slow-rep training. They like it because it helps to camouflage the lack of weight being used. They can always have an excuse for the lack of weight

by saying that they are going slow. Most of the people I know who do slow-rep training never talk about progression, which is why most of them look so puny. Remember, if you do use slow-rep training, the key is still progression regardless of the speed used.

There are exceptions, and more and more strong guys including NFL teams are now using slow-speed training. People like Drew Israel and Jeff Watson train using slow reps, but keep progression as their top priority; and they are getting great results. You do not have to train 10 up and 5 down. Drew is using 10/10; and Jeff Watson has coined "deep training" which is a single rep, or low reps, of 30 seconds or more for each.

95

I'm a regular-speed guy, but still use slow training as a change of pace. At least once a month we will use it. The speed of motion I've been using for this is 8 seconds up and 8 seconds down, for 8 reps to add weight. Slow training is especially good for rehab.

Don't let the so-called experts with narrow definitions of science confuse you. Reread *Brawn* whenever you get confused, and get back to basics. Remember the basic philosophy of hard work, good food, and plenty of recovery time. Combine this with lots of effort and dedication, and you can succeed with one of many specific modes or methods of training.

THE SECOND ANNUAL CAPITAL CITY CLINIC

May 1998

I put out 110 chairs thinking that I should have plenty, but I still had to borrow 6 more from the Chinese restaurant on the first floor. We almost doubled the attendance from last year. A very enthusiastic crowd of 116 people (excluding speakers) showed up, with many having driven hundreds of miles. We had people from all over, including Michigan, Ohio, Ontario, North Carolina, and Colorado. There were many from the New York and New Jersey area, largely because Iron Island Gym was well represented in the speaking department. Probably more than half the crowd was not local.

The theme of this year's clinic was "Elements of Productive Strength Training," and a variety of philosophies was represented by the speakers. My goal was to stress the similarities of all successful training programs, regardless of the specific mode or method used. My view has always been that a good coach can get to the root of things and keep training simple. (People who don't know their subject will frequently hide their lack of knowledge by making things hard to understand.)

Strength training is similar to religion as far as strong opinions go. But by focusing on "getting stronger," and not on minor details, and by stressing the similarities of various philosophies rather than getting into "cat fights," we accomplished a great deal—and all within an atmosphere of brotherhood and camaraderie.

Anyone who did not want this atmosphere of brotherhood and camaraderie was warned that they should keep themselves under control or else they would have to leave. There have been several clinics on the east coast over the last few years that have been disrupted and spoiled by a few individuals who wanted to argue about minor details, and rattle speakers. These individuals say that they are trying to promote their type of training, and "Educate" people, but actually do no more than make people dislike them and reject their ideas. There was a mutual respect for all speakers at the clinic, and a true feeling of brotherhood.

Linda Jo Belsito

Linda Jo, who spoke about drug-free power training and what it takes to be a world champion, is a two-time (and current) world champion drug-free powerlifter (ADFP). She is always up for a new challenge and is now crossing over to Olympic weightlifting. She plans to compete in Olympic lifting soon. Her goal is to make the US Olympic team in the year 2000, in which weightlifting will be open to women for the first time. Linda Jo is stronger than most men, and squats and deadlifts over 400 lbs. She holds many world and national powerlifting records, and works as a Registered Nurse. She has also spent several years working for Dr. Ken at Iron Island Gym.

Linda Jo spoke about her workouts with Dr. Ken, and singled him out as the person who has probably helped her the most during her career. She said that he put her through some absolutely brutal workouts, such as 100-rep days where the only thing in the entire workout was to get 100 reps in the deadlift or squat. She said that those one-exercise workouts were among the toughest things she has ever done in her life.

Like many women, she used to be worried about her weight. Dr. Ken told her that if she was going to get stronger and be a champion powerlifter, she was going to have to eat. She would have to decide between bodybuilding and powerlifting. She decided to go into powerlifting. Her bodybuilding days were over. (She had previously been competing at bodybuilding, winning some amateur titles.) Once she focused on getting stronger, and eating what her body needed rather than be obsessed with a number on the scale, her poundages went way up!

98

She made up her mind that she was going to be a champion, and improved the details of her life that make a difference. She focused on getting more sleep each night, and eating better, and stopped partying. She started to really believe in herself, stopped associating with negative people, bought and read a lot of positive-thinking books, and listened to positive-thinking tapes.

Drew Israel

Drew Israel did more to advance slow training with his awesome demonstration of strength than all the cat fights ever did! Drew did several 10/10 gut-wrenching reps (ten seconds up, and ten seconds down) till he looked as if he was struck by lightning. He did this with well over 400 lbs on my Hammer Deadlift machine. Most people can't do one rep with that using a regular speed, never mind a 10/10 cadence. Drew also did slow prone presses and upright rows on the same machine. Shortly afterwards he did some manual resistance work, with Eric Weinstein providing the resistance. Because Drew deadlifted first, and did not stay down long to recover, he was breathing extremely hard, which made the rest of his workout a lot tougher than it may sound on paper. The deadlifts alone were a workout and most people would have been KOed after doing them as hard as Drew did.

Drew spoke about how he made many training mistakes over the years. He has tried many training methods, and suffered many injuries. He especially had trouble with his back, and had to give up squatting with a barbell many years ago. He now trains almost exclusively with machines (no free weights except for an occasional set of dumbbell curls,) and works his legs with the Tru-Squat, Hammer Deadlift, and Hammer Leg Press. He started using slow-cadence training about a year and a half ago, and found it very beneficial for him. He loves it and now only trains using a slow cadence.

Drew does not like the image that many people have of training using slow reps, i.e., that it is only for wimps. It absolutely is not for wimps as it is a lot of hard work, and painful. Since he began to train slow, he now hardly ever gets hurt, and his body recovers a lot quicker than it did with conventional speed reps. Drew also feels that slow training is making him stronger than he has ever been.

Eric Weinstein & Jamie La Belle

Eric, featured in my "Nightmare on Seventh Street" article in issue #52, was put through a tough workout by Drew. Eric's workout was finished off by two trips around the large room (and crowd) with the 225-lb sandbag. He got a thunderous ovation, as people appreciate hard work.

Classic high-intensity training was well represented by myself and Jamie La Belle. My talk was very similar to the information in my article in issue #53, in which I described intensity as the unifying factor.

Jamie trains many professional athletes in all sports, and is a big believer in the importance of balanced routines and not overlooking any muscle group. He puts a lot of emphasis on the neck, wrists, calves, ankles and abs, which are undertrained areas for many athletes. He made a great point when he stated, "How many NFL players got put out of action by hurting their chests?" But the chest is usually the most overworked area. Most injuries are of the forgotten areas, which Jamie focused on.

Jamie stressed that most people spend too much time bench pressing. As a result they do not spend enough time on the exercises needed to keep their strength in balance over their whole body. Jamie usually has to train someone with twice as many pulling exercises as pushing exercises because they are so out of whack due to having spent so much time on the bench.

Jamie has his athletes do a lot of rowing, pulldowns and chins. He also uses a lot of manual resistance work, and is able to apply this for every muscle of the body. He has special manual resistance exercises to work even ankles, and has devised a manual resistance squat, which is a killer. He loves to pre-exhaust muscles, especially for very strong athletes with big egos who have their minds only on big numbers.

Jamie frequently takes the bench press out of his athletes' workouts, to get their training in proper balance. And when he does include the bench press, he will frequently have his athletes do it at the end of the workout, after their chests and triceps have already been hammered. Then the athletes are forced to get their minds off numbers and just on working hard.

Jamie uses mostly machines as opposed to free weights, in his well-equipped gym on Long Island. He has machines that cover the neck, calves and abs. He trains these small areas using the same principles employed for the big areas. He uses a slower-than-average speed of motion for all his machine exercises—about six seconds up and six seconds down. He stops his athletes from completely locking out, to keep a constant tension on the muscles. He is a big believer in the one-set-to-total-failure principle, but uses such a variety of exercises that his total volume for a workout would not be considered low. But keep in mind that he focuses on training competitive athletes. Jamie is highly opposed to ballistic type explosive training, especially plyometrics.

Andrea Rippe & Jay Spaid

Andrea Rippe, who was featured in my "Dinosaur Women" article in issue #46, gave a great talk about exercise selection and the importance of using compound multi-joint exercises as the foundation of your training program, similar to one of the themes of *Brawn*. She talked a lot about the balance between high volume and high intensity, and that if you do the hardest exercises intensively you can cut your volume way down. Many people spend too much time in the gym, but not enough time really working.

Jay Spaid gave a good talk about recovery. He coined the five- and six-day-per-week program as "drug routines," and used some advertisements and articles from muscle mags to show the absurdity of much of the popular modern training routines.

One of our planned speakers, Brooks Kubik, who is a lawyer by trade, did not attend. He called just a few hours before the start of the clinic, to advise that he had a work-related "legal emergency" to attend to. It didn't matter, as each speaker talked a bit longer than planned, and we even covered his topic, the mental aspects of training. The clinic actually ran about thirty minutes over, and went to 3:30 p.m.

This was a hands-on clinic—a coaches' clinic, not a researchers' clinic. We did not talk about actin and myosin, or the sliding-filament theory. We did not talk about how to organize a weightroom, periodization of synchronized swimmers, NSCA budgets or elections, or other boring typical clinic topics. We focused on the "meat and potatoes" of training. We focused on passion and the love of training that bonds us, not boring, "scientific" statistics to "prove" a point of view, and divide. We focused on strength training, not "conditioning." When I opened the clinic with, "I'd like to welcome you to the second annual Capital City

National Strength and Conditioning Association clinic," I shouted "Strength" but whispered "Conditioning," to make the focus of the clinic clear. Strength training is what most people want, and why I had so many people say that this was the best NSCA clinic they had ever attended.

One of the funny things that happened during the clinic was when a pigeon few in an open window and flew around the room. when it tried to fly out, it flew into a pane of glass and fell to the floor. Jamie La Belle yelled "PLYOMETRICS!" just as the pigeon fell to the floor. Luckily the pigeon was okay, just stunned. A few minutes later, the pigeon did the same thing again, and in unison many of the audience yelled "PLYOMETRICS!"

COMMANDO-TOUGH INTENSITY

July 1998

Saturday is my favorite day to go to work. I have a great line up of hard-working athletes coming in. Athletes are my favorite clients to train because I can let out all stops and pull no punches. On Saturdays it's like a conveyor belt bringing in guys who pay me to level them! One after the other they keep coming in and keep getting laid out. We usually do sandbag on Saturday, too, as people are not in a hurry like they usually are on other days. I can also sleep late and have a big brunch. I'm usually up at 5AM each day during the week and work a morning and evening shift. On Saturday I work one non-stop shift, from noon to 7 PM.

I arrived an hour early and set up the plates on the machines, filled the water bottles and loaded the sandbags. I went over each client's training records and logged the day's planned workout for each client, wrote down poundages, etc., so that when we are in the heat of battle I won't have to waste time looking for poundages, etc.

I had the Masimini brothers, Themba and Mpumi (pronounced "Timba" and "Poomie") coming in back to back, followed by Melvin Tuten and Joe Bunton. Themba, 22, is 6'4'' and 270 pounds. He's a recent graduate of Howard University where he played tight end for four years on the football team. He was one of the final cuts of the Baltimore Ravens last summer. He's training to make the NFL this year and has been invited to try out by three teams. Themba jokingly calls Mpumi his "little" brother when he really means his younger brother. Mpumi is 20 and a junior at Howard. He's an offensive tackle on the football team, and is 6'4'' and 315 pounds. Some little brother! And some genetics!

Themba is a friend of Melvin Tuten. Big Melvin had to twist Themba's arm to get him to train with me. Melvin even paid for Themba's first workout, and wanted me to hammer him. Melvin had been telling Themba about his training and how Themba

103

should sign up. Themba was skeptical, as many people are, when he heard about training "only two hours a week" with weights. He probably thought it was not enough and that it wasn't tough. Melvin paid to give Themba the "experience." After his first workout Themba totally changed his mind. Then he paid for his brother's first workout, and came to watch me hammer Mpumi. Mpumi, too, has changed his way of thinking. The experience of a brutal workout will change an opinion a lot faster and better than trying to explain it. If you haven't been through it, you just don't understand.

The Workouts

Brutal strength-training workouts burn a lot of calories. You can't train when you are out of fuel, and your body can't compensate for poor fuel. All my clients have a 300-400 calorie high-carbohydrate snack about two hours before training. Themba had a bowl of pasta at 11AM and arrived at around 1PM. He was breathing steam and ready to kick some ass! I put him on the Stairmaster for five minutes to "pre-heat" his muscles and elevate his core body temperature. Then he did a series of twenty-second static hold stretches, and a series of warmup sets with the machines to be used.

Many of my clients are friends, and come in to watch workouts and root their friends on. Big Melvin just came in with Mpumi, and shouted encouragement to Themba over the blasting cadence tape.

Themba started off with the Hammer Chest Press and went to failure, doing 9 reps with 270 pounds. I quickly pulled off two 45-pound plates and Themba immediately went to failure again, with 180 pounds. When he hit failure I stripped off two more 45s and he went to failure again, this time with a ten-second static hold at the end of the set. Then we moved to pullovers.

Themba went to failure on the Hammer Pullover machine with 180 pounds, holding the crossbar on his waist for a "one-one thousand hold" at the bottom of each rep. The pullover is an exercise in which good form plays a huge part in determining effectiveness. I used to allow clients to just touch their waists with the crossbar, and it looked like they were drilling for oil. I only recently bought this machine and am still learning about the best way to use it. After speaking with Dr. Ken about it, I decided to insist on the dead stop pause with the crossbar against the user's waist, and to make this possible I decreased everyone's poundages by about 50 pounds. This stricter form makes a huge difference for hitting the lats and not just the rear delts. Themba was using about 240 pounds when he was "drilling for oil," now he's howling with just 180! After Themba went to failure with 180 I broke down the machine twice, and added a ten-second static hold.

Next was the dumbbell curl with 2-inch diameter handles. He went to failure with 50-pound dumbbells and I added a few forced reps at the end of the set. He was now dripping in sweat and the droplets were raining on the floor. After a short rest it was over to the Nautilus Power Plus Military Press with 180 pounds. After hitting failure at 11 reps I broke it down to 135 and he went to failure again. I then switched the machine from isolateral to bilateral mode, and gave him some forced reps and a ten-second static hold.

The Tru-Squat was next, everyone's favorite! Themba eked out 23 reps with 190 pounds and had to go down on one knee and then lay on the floor for a few minutes after the set. He was drenched in sweat and breathing like a steam engine. After another rest and some water, he felt okay and was anxious to finish.

The final challenge of the day was the farmer's walk around the block with 100-pound dumbbells. Melvin, Mpumi and myself served as escorts, guiding Themba through the congested streets.

We cleared the streets ahead of Themba. It took about twenty minutes to get him around the block as Themba had to put the dumbbells down about fifteen times to make it. His shoulders, lats, forearms and hands were just destroyed! He was "stress free" when he completed the walk—so wiped out that he could not feel any discomfort, or have any worries.

Melvin and Mpumi went through workouts similar to Themba's. Today was "breakdown day" but we don't do breakdowns all the time. It's just something we do once in a while.

Hard Training at 47 Years Young

Everyone talks about training hard, but the definition of hard will depend on the person. Hard for a beginner in his forties will not be the same as hard for an athlete in his twenties. I see a wide variety of people at Whelan Strength Training. Most of the people I train are in their twenties and thirties, but I also have some in their forties and fifties. I also have several women who train using the same principles of progression and intensity as the men.

One of my hardest workers is 47 years young—"Big Daddy" Joe Bunton. Joe is not an athlete but I almost view him as one because he trains extremely hard. Joe has transformed himself in the last two years. When Joe first came to me he was living in the seventies. He was overweight, on medication for high blood pressure, was listening to 20-year-old disco music, and had a Don-King-like "grey Afro." Joe works at a cemetery and sees funerals every day. One of the reasons why he started training was because he didn't want to be a "customer" at the cemetery any time soon.

Joe is now a lot stronger and a lot leaner. He's off the medication, shaved his head, and listens to rap music! I keep telling Joe that he's not aging. He's youthing!

Joe was quiet and almost timid when he started training. Finally, after a few weeks of trying to get Joe excited, I asked him what got him really mad. Joe mentioned several things, most of them related to racial issues. For the next several weeks I would yell those thing at him whenever Joe did leg presses, deadlifts or Tru-Squats. But after each workout Joe used to thank me for getting him so charged up. He got so excited that he made the weights look light. His poundages shot way up. I now no longer have to yell at him to get

106

him charged up. His mind is trained. Now he's the most focused, ferocious, loudest client I have!

Joe even does the sandbag carry and is almost at the point of mastering 175 pounds at "sandbag alley." If someone is way out of shape, or over 40, we don't even think about the sandbag until the person has spent several months training with me, and has proven him/herself. I trained Joe for several months before he tried it, but now Joe trains harder than most young guys.

Consistency is the key. Keep strength training regularly, and keep doing your cardio-vascular training. Enjoy your training, and look forward to your workouts. Training hard should be enjoyed. If you truly enjoy training, you will reap your just share of rewards.

TRAINING STRATEGIES

September 1998

It takes most people about three weeks of working out at Whelan Strength Training before they are able to complete my one-hour planned workout. Some take longer, and some such as young well-conditioned athletes will come along a lot quicker.

Once they have completed the initial conditioning phase and are able to perform the planned work, my number one goal as coach is to get them through it every time. I would be hurting their training if I flattened them before all the training at any given workout was done. Knocking someone out early in a workout is easy—the human body can only take so much. Any coach can do that, but a good coach tries to get each trainee through the entire workout. That's the hard part. If a trainee goes down, I want him or her back up in a few minutes, to finish. I really want my charges to stay on their feet till the end of each workout. I want to push them to the edge of the cliff, but not over it till the work is all done. If they stay down after the last planned set, that's okay because they have finished the work.

Achieving this requires different techniques for different people. Some need an extra minute of rest at a few points during the workout. Some need positive strokes, and some need a kick in the ass. Some like or need a lot of shouting, and some don't. Some need a goal drilled into their head. They need a target because they have trouble thinking in terms of "going to failure." I usually give such trainees a high number that would be hard to reach, so they will go to failure. But they need a number, just like a "smart bomb" needs a chimney and not just a building.

Other people don't want to know the weight on the bar or have any knowledge of their previous best performances for reps, because this puts pressure on them. I lie a lot to these people. I'll tell them the wrong weight (usually that it's lighter) or don't tell them the weight or reps until they are done. I frequently give them wrong information on purpose so they won't know what to expect. My goal with them is to take the pressure off. Some people respond well to pressure and some don't. It's the coach's job to learn what motivates each athlete. The coach should still push to get the best out of each trainee, but use a different mental technique in doing so, when necessary.

Exercise Sequence

Exercise sequence is a big factor in the success of many of my clients. Many people cannot do justice to the rest of their workout if they do legs first. Do not get hung up on absolute rules such as "always work larger muscles first." That is just a general guideline. There are other less popular theories of exercise sequence such as pre-exhaustion, which is usually the opposite of working the largest muscles first. And there is the bodybuilding philosophy of work out the weakest body part first, or working first the parts of the physique that need the most improvement, in order to bring about symmetry. Exercise sequence varies from individual to individual and boils down to performance strategy.

You'll usually do better at what you do first or at the beginning of a workout, but you don't want to do anything first that greatly alters (or *ends*) the rest of the workout. The philosophy of working the largest muscles first is good in theory *and* in practice for many people, but for some it's a disaster. When training for "general fitness" it's easy to train the larger muscles first, but for really intensive training a few hard sets of deadlifts or squats could mean *lights out* for many trainees—workout over!

This is especially true when doing multiple sets. Remember that many "larger muscles first" advocates (who train in a high-intensity fashion) usually do just one set to failure per exercise. Single set training to failure is tough, but two or three sets to failure for a lower-body exercise is suicidal for many people if done at the beginning of a workout. If you do multiple sets and feel impaired after doing legs first in a workout, try doing legs at the end of your workout. Your upper body will thank you for it.

You are also supposed to enjoy your training. If you *like* to do legs first, fine. But if it's agony for you and impairs the rest of your workout, don't do it.

My number one goal as a coach is to get my charges through the planned workout. I don't want them to do just squats and be done. I also don't want them to be impaired to the point that they are weak in upper-body exercises because they are so wiped out. I've found that upper-body exercises don't affect the lower-body exercises nearly as much as vice versa. Many if not most of my charges do their squats, deadlifts and leg presses after everything else is done. That way, if they go down and are KOed, it's the end of the workout and everything else has already been done, so nothing gets sacrificed.

Alternate Push and Pull

A rule that I follow is using an equal number of pushing and pulling exercises at each workout. I usually perform a pushing and a pulling exercise for the horizontal and vertical planes for the upper body at each workout, and rotate the leg press, deadlift and Tru-Squat. (This may, however, be too much for some people. You may respond better to training the horizontal and vertical planes just once a week each.) For some advanced trainees I employ the Hammer Deadlift and Leg Press at the same workout, e.g., see Thursday's workout (on page 21).

It's a good idea to alternate the pushing and pulling exercises so there is built-in recovery between exercises even though you are not actually resting. You'll lose too much strength if you do multiple pushing or pulling exercises back to back, e.g., overhead press followed by the bench press. I usually have my charges perform three exercises in a row with no rest between sets, and then have them take a minute off. If there is a leg exercise in the group (squat, leg press or deadlift) it will be put last in the group of three exercises. If there are two leg exercises in the same workout, a longer rest is allowed after the leg exercise in the first grouping.

Change-of-Pace Days

I'm a big believer in employing a "strategic" change-of-pace day once in a while. Mixing up your training is helpful and makes exercise fun. It's also plain smart. When you establish certain traditions on certain days of the month or year you really look forward to those special days, and get motivated. Motivation is the key to training success. The main three change-of-pace days I use are fifties day (several to-failure sets per exercise that add up to 50 reps, e.g., 15, 12, 10, 7, 6), breakdown day (e.g., to failure, strip off weight, more reps to failure, and then another cut in poundage and a final string of reps), and slow-cadence day.

Motivation is also developed by the sandbag and farmer's walk. In my experience people will "kill" themselves just to get their name put on the bag. I've had people drive five hours to Washington, DC, just to try to get their name put on the bag, or to try the "walk of doom" around the block in downtown DC with 100-pound dumbbells.

When you mix it up, remember that this strategy is still part of the overall plan, so it's not haphazard. I'll go two or three weeks and have a planned change of pace day. These days incorporate the same exercises that would have been done on that day, but performed in a different manner to usual—usually fifties day, breakdown fashion, or very slow cadence. Because this is planned, I'll check back to the last day the same special workout was performed, and provide goals (or lie about the poundages) for those who need it.

Example core program

Monday
     1. Bench Press /Horizontal Tru-Press: 3 x 8
     2. Seated Cable Row /Hammer Iso-Lateral Row: 3 x 8
     3. Shoulder Shrug: 3 x 15

4. Military Press: 3 x 8
5. Pulldowns: 3 x 8
6. Squats: 2 x 20

Thursday
1. Incline Press /Hammer Chest Press: 3 x 8
2. Pullovers: 3 x 10
3. Deadlifts: 2 x 10
3-4 minutes rest after the deadlift
4. Dips: 3 x 10
5. Dumbbell Curl: 3 x 8
6. Leg Press: 2 x 20

On change-of-pace days, we usually don't perform shrugs or curls.

Warmup sets are additional to the sets listed above. For both core workouts, "finishers," which include the sandbag carry, farmer's walk and grip work, are performed at the end of each session, time and energy permitting.

Do not use change-of-pace days too often. Stay the course for at least two or three weeks on your core workouts before you inject a change-of-pace session. If you are over forty, or a beginner, think twice about fifties days. They should be reserved for young athletes and trainees in very good shape who enjoy this sort of grueling challenge. But even for them, fifties days or other types of extreme high-rep work should not be performed more than once a month. Some people, however, should never do this sort of training because it's too grueling for them.

I would not make changes to the overall core plan (i.e., core workouts interspersed with a change-of-pace session every few weeks) for at least 3-4 months. Give it time to work and time for you to learn from it. Forget the micro-cycle nonsense. Keep good records—write down everything and learn from your records. After 3-4 months, try some changes. Try different exercises, rep ranges or even speed of motion if you are so inclined. Don't be afraid to experiment *sensibly.* (Do not ALWAYS do 20-rep squats.) Train for 3-4 months using one rep range and then 3-4 months using another rep range. Find what works best for you. Enjoy your training and train smarter as well as harder.

Mental Training

As I've mentioned in other articles, I strongly encourage my clients to read motivational/positive thinking books, and listen to motivational cassette tapes. The world is largely *negative.* The more positive reinforcement, the better. Learning how to think like a champion will have a big impact on your training and life in general. I especially recommend *The Magic of Thinking Big* by David Schwartz. Order it from BobWhelan.com. You can get motivational tapes from Nightingale Conant, 7300 North Lehigh Avenue, Niles, IL 60714, USA. I especially recommend *The Psychology of Winning* by Dennis Waitley, but anything from Zig Zigler, Norman Vincent Peale, Og Mandino, Tony Robbins or Robert Schuller is also very good. You can order almost anything from BobWhelan.com's amazon store.

Nutritional Strategy

Beware of "nutritionists" (who are not registered dieticians) and personal trainers who give nutritional advice. Never take the advice of minimum-wage clerks who work in health food stores. Consult only a registered dietician. One of the most respected RDs in the world is Nancy Clark. She is the nutritional consultant to the Boston Red Sox and Boston Celtics. She offers seminars, books and various helpful nutritional flyers that are the *real deal,* not the latest hype. A link to her site can be found on NaturalStrength.com

CHAMPIONS HAVE THE WILL TO SUCCEED

November 1998

A few months ago I got a phone call from Matt Brzycki, strength and conditioning coach at Princeton University. Matt wanted me to train one of his athletes for the summer. Jamie Sullivan is from suburban Maryland, right outside Washington, D.C., and needed some hard training to stay in top shape for when he returns to Princeton in September. I was more than happy to accommodate Jamie.

Jamie is a member of the Princeton lacrosse team. Princeton University is the current (and three-time) NCAA national champion in lacrosse. Princeton is to lacrosse what Notre Dame and Penn State are to football. Jamie plays lacrosse year round. Success seems to follow him, as his summer league team won the championship in its league.

More than a few times, Jamie had a summer league game on the same day he had a brutal workout with me. Jamie did not want an easier workout though. I hammered him and pulled no punches. We did everything including the sandbag carry, even on game days. He was still able to play all out even after being hammered earlier in the day. Oh to be young!

A Summer of Preparation

Jamie focused resolutely on his main goal—to be ready and stronger for Princeton in the fall. Jamie only needs to be told things once. He listens, is polite, and works very hard. I tell him what to do, and he does it. I told him to buy motivational books and tapes, and he did it. I told him to eat a big breakfast, lunch and dinner, three snacks (e.g., a can or two of tuna, turkey or chicken per snack), 5-9 servings of fruit and vegetables per day, and drink up

114

to a half gallon of skim milk per day. He didn't make excuses about why he couldn't do it. He did it.

Jamie has to be a bright kid to go to Princeton, and it shows. I gave him a copy of *Brawn* and a few other books to read, and he read them all in just a few days. I quizzed him on the material just to make sure he really read it, and he had! I gave him the same two-hour orientation that I give all my "regular" clients. He was extremely attentive and took notes even though I gave him several pages of handouts that covered the material. I could tell right away that Jamie would get good results because of his excellent attitude.

Jamie followed the same training program I outlined in the last issue, with one exception. In early August we started doing one-legged deadlifts on the Hammer Deadlift machine, instead of using two legs. Hammer Strength recently made a conversation piece to install on the back of the machine that allows you to place the non-lifting leg there to keep your balance. It's even harder than the regular two-legged deadlift. In fact, some of my clients hate it even more than the Tru-Squat! The first use of the one-legged deadlift can produce glute and hamstrings soreness that lasts a week. Dr. Ken and Drew Israel got their conversion pieces a few weeks earlier, and just raved about them. They told me, "Bob, you have to get this!" They were not exaggerating. My clients don't seem to appreciate my talking to Dr. Ken, because he's always giving me ideas to make their workouts even harder!

Crucial Details and the Will to Succeed

Most champions have the willingness to adhere strictly to crucial details like not partying too much, cutting down on or eliminating alcohol, getting enough sleep, maintaining a positive attitude, and especially keeping quality nutrition a top priority. This is why Jamie has gained 16 pounds of muscle and a lot of strength over the summer. He has gone from 158 pounds to 174 while keeping his bodyfat at around 12%. Jamie has the desire and will to succeed, which are the qualities that make a true champion.

115

The cause of failure for many people is that they don't pay attention to vital details that can make all the difference. A huge factor in the success or failure of young college athletes is alcohol. Many of these athletes will do everything right except this part, and then wonder why they are not making the gains that they should. For these youngsters, if they are drinking and out late more than once a week, they can forget about getting good results and getting into top shape. Older trainees, and all hard gainers, can't afford even one very late night each week if they are serious about gaining well. Young and gifted athletes can break some of the rules and get away with it. Hard gainers can't. Alcohol abuse will ruin recovery ability, and ruin chances of getting bodyfat down. Alcohol use is the Achilles heel of many training programs, and the missing link in the success of many people. Coaches need to give this a lot more attention.

A large percentage of my current clients are athletes. A few are professional, but most are college athletes, with some in high school. They are my favorite clients to train because they are usually already hungry to improve, and have very specific goals. Non-athletes can learn from the behavior of disciplined athletes. Though non-athletes usually do not have the youth and natural talent of the athletes, they can still learn from them.

Pervis Ellison is back for a second summer of high-intensity training. He had a great first half of the season last year. He was named a captain by coach Pitino, and the Boston media was raving about his physical improvement. He seemed to be on the way to the comeback of the year when he suffered another bad injury during a basketball game. Hopefully Pervis will have better luck this year.

I also have a third Masimini as a client. The "boys" have a sister named Thande, who is 6-4 and 200 pounds! She plays professional basketball. Her two brothers escorted her in for a few workouts and encouraged me to train her real hard while they watched. She is currently playing for a team in France.

116

The high school athletes are especially fun to train because they are so eager to learn. They are easy to motivate and usually can be trained extremely hard right off the bat. They pay attention to the important details and don't fluff anything off, especially with their parents paying for the training. The key thing, however, is that they have the will to succeed and are determined to get results come hell or high water. This makes my job a lot easier. Anyone can have this will to achieve, regardless of age or responsiveness to training.

The discipline to do what it takes, in and out of the gym, is what's needed to get maximum results. There will be plateaus, sticking points and frustration, of course. It's like that for everyone, though some people suffer more than others.

It's the special will to succeed that separates the achievers from the underachievers. The achievers are more than willing to put out the effort that it takes to get results. Their minds are positive and they refuse to accept failure. They have positive self talk which is extremely important. When they have a disappointing set in terms of the number of reps performed, they don't whine and say negative things about themselves, or what a bad day they are having. They just believe they will be stronger next time and go to the next machine with the "eye of the tiger" and their mental focus unchanged. They channel their anger into a better performance on the next set, and do not waste energy in a negative manner.

One of my goals as coach is to channel anger and frustration in a positive way. Anger and frustration are great sources of energy. Learning how to channel this energy positively is vital for maximizing your potential.

I can tell by the noise my clients make while they train whether or not they are using positive or negative energy. If they sound angry and vicious when they train—like a wild lion roaring—I know they are in the proper mind set. But if they make a whining, moaning sort of sound, I know they are in a negative mode. Some highly focused and motivated people train without making much noise, as noted by Dr. Ken in issue #55, but the noise they make is still the "right" type.

When someone is in negative mode, I usually immediately end the set and give him/her a lecture on the spot about how the mind must be in gear to train, or else it's better to go home and not even bother. You need all the energy you can muster when training hard. You can't train productively if your mind is in negative mode.

Many of my non-athlete clients don't have this proper mental attitude right away. I stay hard on them and don't smile or act friendly to them until they have developed the proper mental attitude. It is usually someone's lack of positive expectations and selling themselves short at the start of training that is the biggest obstacle for me to overcome. Once they start to think properly, then at least they are giving themselves the chance to get results. If they have a negative attitude, however, they have no chance.

Age is Only a Number

I am 44 years old, but am told by many people that I look and act at least ten years younger. This can make things interesting.

Frequently, new non-athlete clients only in their mid to late thirties come in with a negative attitude and say things like, "When I was your age I could train hard and do squats and deadlifts, but you've got to remember that I'm 37 years old!" I usually get a good laugh and tell them that they are "still in puberty," or "you still need acne medicine."

The first thing I do is change their outlook and attitude about training, or encourage them to train somewhere else. I believe that there are two types of age: chronological age that you can't do anything about but which is only a number, and biological age that you can do something about. I keep telling the older guys that by training they are "youthing," not aging.

Keep your expectations realistically high and don't sell yourself short. Of course it may take a while to build up your conditioning and strength safely, but what matters most is that you make a start and believe in improvement. The mind—through having positive expectations and a positive attitude—is by far the most important factor determining training success. Pay close attention to major factors such as alcohol use, sleep and nutrition that could be your Achilles heel. It is, however, the lack of a positive attitude that is usually responsible for not paying attention to the crucial details. With the right attitude you will get all the details in good order.

YOU'RE NOT AGING...YOU'RE YOUTHING!

January 1999

*"Age is a question of mind over matter. If you
don't mind, it doesn't matter."*
— Satchel Paige

"Getting older is not for sissies."
—Jack Palance

There's no such thing as the fountain of youth, but strength training is the closest thing to it. Strength training is no longer thought of as only a hobby of youth, but a lifetime endeavor. In fact, it gets even more important as you get older. Cardiovascular training is vital, and everyone should be doing it regularly—at least three times per week—but *in addition* to strength training. If you only do cardiovascular training you may live to be 90 years old, but you'll more than likely look and feel old for the last 40 years of your life.

Cardiovascular training gives you the "quantity of life," but strength training gives you the "quality of life." Without strength training you'll probably still struggle to carry your groceries, you could fall and break your hip, and have the same age-related problems of lean muscle tissue loss, bone density loss (osteoporosis), arthritis and lack of strength that other senior citizens have.

Have you ever stood at the end of the marathon race, and watched the runners come in? Even though they are accomplishing a tremendous physical feat, most of them (who don't lift weights) look like hell. Other than being trim, the older runners look no different than any untrained older person. After they shower, change and put their business suits back on, they will look ordinary, and most people won't believe that they even completed the race. Cardiovascular training alone will not come close to retarding the aging process. You'll just end up with a healthy heart in an average body.

Every year, more and more research information is coming in about the benefits of "strength training for life," and the news is good. In fact, some of the latest research states that strength training is now considered at least as important as cardiovascular training for overall health, with some studies claiming it's even more important, especially when you get older. A big reason for this is that many people are unable to move much at all when they get older. Strength training liberates them to be able to do cardiovascular exercise and other things in order to lead independent lives.

Most of my clients are in their twenties and thirties, but I've some older ones who are dedicated and train very hard. You've previously read about "Big Daddy" Joe Bunton, who went from "grey afro" to shaved head, disco to rap, and off the high blood pressure medication. He looks about fifteen years younger than when he started, and is in such good shape that I let him do the sandbag carry at age 47, without fear of him dropping. I also have other older high achievers like him.

Frank Farrow

Frank Farrow is in his early fifties but is tenacious, with great mental focus—sometimes too great. He is one of the best I've ever seen, regardless of age, at truly going to muscular failure. Frank seemed to understand the concept right away and took to it like a duck to water . He is the only person for whom I have to end many of the sets because he wants to persist until he ends up looking like a "tortured, vibrating sack of isometrics." In one of his first workouts with me he was doing shrugs and kept going 'til the weight totally stopped moving. But he didn't stop, and was shaking, grimacing, growling, breathing like a steam engine, and dripping with sweat for another 20 seconds doing what looked to be isometrics. I watched with amazement and finally had to make him stop.

When people first call me about training, I don't sugar coat anything. I lay out my philosophy plain for everyone to see regardless of age. Many people get scared off, but that's okay because we would probably not be a good match anyway. Training with me is not a democracy, but I don't turn away anyone who is determined to join the program and follow my instruction. I don't care if they have trained before, or are beginners. I don't care about their gender or age. All I require is a philosophical match. If they are willing to work as they have never worked before, are not looking for gimmicks, and want to maximize their natural, genetic potential for muscular development, strength and overall body stamina and fitness, then we will get along great.

Art Brown

Recently, Art Brown called me. Art is 63 years old and was not in great shape. He had never exercised in his life and didn't know anything about training. All Art knew was that he felt weak, old and unhealthy, and wanted to make some changes. I came on strong with Art but he was not scared off, and had a great attitude. He put his trust completely in my hands. Even though Art is by far my oldest client, I was happy to help him. Frank Farrow used to be my oldest client, but Art jokingly calls Frank "sonny boy" now. I had to start Art slow. I mean s-l-o-w! For the first month I mainly built up Art's cardiovascular conditioning and overall fitness, doing mostly Stairmaster, ab work, stretching and a very short weight workout. My main goal was just to keep him alive through the one-hour workout.

After a month, Art was able to perform 30 minutes on the Stairmaster fairly easily, so I weaned him into more strength training and gradually let him do the cardio work in his own time. I have to admit that the first few workouts with Art were scary. I made him take long rests between sets for the first month or so, and made sure that he did not breathe too hard. I would tell him,

"Breathe deeply, Art, but above all, breathe!" He could only go down one hole on the Tru-Squat, with no weight, and used many other machines with a very light weight to start with.

Art has now been training for about three months and has doubled his strength on most exercises, and now goes to the bottom on the Tru-Squat for 10 reps. He has greatly increased his range of motion in many exercises. He noticeably suffered from arthritis when he started, but now the arthritis does not bother him. He acts and feels ten years younger already!

The main motivation for Art to train was his work. He works in the National Science Foundation, a branch of the US Government. He specializes in polar operations, and spent the first twenty years of his career going to the North Pole area and Greenland, and he's spent around the last twenty years making trips to the South Pole area (Antarctica). The last few trips have been rough and he has literally almost been blown away (or frozen) a few times, and he has barely passed the physical required. Art is one of just a few men who have gone to both the North and South Pole. He's making another Antarctica trip soon, and recently passed his physical with flying colors. His doctors were amazed, and told him his physical data had not looked this good in over ten years.

Vic Boff and Joe Marino

Vic and Joe are friends of mine, and are in phenomenal shape for their ages. Vic is in his eighties and is one of the all-time legends in physical culture. He still trains regularly and hard, and looks and acts twenty years younger than his age. Vic does not let age slow him down at all. Joe Marino is in his sixties and trains as hard as ever. Joe competed in a lot of major bodybuilding contests in the fifties, winning several titles. Joe is very fit and still as enthusiastic and dedicated to his training as ever. He puts most younger guys to shame. Vic and Joe have an abundance of energy and enthusiasm, and an endless supply of physical culture stories from the glory days long past when there were no such things as steroids. Vic was a good friend of both George Jowett and Sig Klein, and Joe was a long-time training partner and still a close friend of Marvin Elder.

Vic and Joe visited me recently, at Whelan Strength Training, and we had a great time. The three of us, together with my girlfriend, Sue, had dinner later, and talked so much that it was like going back in time.

It's Never Too Late to Start

Dr. William Evans, Chief of the Human Physiology Laboratory at the USDA Human Nutrition Research Center on Aging at Tufts University in Boston has spent a lifetime studying aging and the benefits of strength training. In a *USA Today* interview, Dr. Evans states, "There is nothing like a lifetime of physical activity to help prevent a whole host of chronic diseases. Starting early on is important...but it's never too late to begin. Our oldest subject is 101 years old. He's been lifting weights for four years. He's probably as strong as a typical man who is forty years his junior but who doesn't exercise...Much of the loss of muscle with age is preventable...We can make a 70-year-old man stronger than he has ever been in his life. We can bring back strength and aerobic capacity. We can make people thinner and reduce their bodyfat levels."

Personally, I'm stronger now than I've ever been. It's really true that you don't lose strength for decades longer than previously thought. It just takes more thought and discipline to maintain conditioning and avoid injury. I now need a longer warmup and more stretching, and more rest and recovery than I used to. But once I'm warmed up, especially my elbows, I can lift more than ever. I also need less food and more cardiovascular work than I used to. I used to be able to eat anything and everything, but now, if I'm not careful and disciplined, I can gain bodyfat very easily.
Everyone needs to make adjustments as they get older, but the basic philosophy remains the same. The rewards are great, as strength training, probably more than anything, helps keep you young. Strength training, just like brushing your teeth, should be a lifetime activity.

JOHN GRIMEK WAS "THE MAN"

March 1999

For all of my training life I've had the quiet comfort of knowing John Grimek was around to inspire and motivate me. He was my all-time Iron Game hero, a legend of unparalleled achievements, but who was universally described as a "good guy" by everyone who had the honor of meeting him. He was a guy you could really admire, look up to and respect not only for his titles or measurements, but as a man.

His pictures have always been on the walls of my gym even if it happened to be my bedroom or garage. I have several of his pictures on the walls at Whelan Strength Training, from various decades of his life starting with the Mark Berry posters showing John in his early twenties, until several decades later showing his body even more muscular and better, with only his face showing signs of age. For my money, he was the best, a legend—*the man!* This greatest chapter in Iron Game history came to a close on November 20, 1998 when John C. Grimek passed on at age 88.

Vic Boff summed it up well when he stated, "For over five decades, John C. Grimek has been heralded as the Monarch of Muscledom throughout the world. He was the greatest combination Iron Game athlete—physique star, bodybuilder and strength performer—of all time and certainly the most popular, inspiring millions. He was a major influence in the lives of every top bodybuilder. He was the only bodybuilder in history who was never defeated in a contest. His charisma was so outstanding that everyone in the Iron Game wanted to meet him, shake his hand or get an autograph. His obliging patience was endless."

Grimek was also the only man to win the Mr. America title twice, and was also a member of the 1936 US Olympic weightlifting team. He won the Mr. Universe in 1948 and the Mr. USA in 1949.

He was also an expert swimmer, diver, acrobat and muscle control expert. He was also very strong, and capable of a 400-pound jerk.

John probably did more to advance strength training in academia, teaching and coaching than anyone—especially as a legitimate method for training and preparing athletes. The all-prevalent musclebound myths of the day were largely dispelled and reversed by his awesome demonstrations of flexibility, grace and speed while working with Bob Hoffman and other members of the York Barbell Club. Modern strength and conditioning coaches may not have had a profession if not for John C. Grimek.

I began to train, involuntarily at first, at age 10. I was a good baseball player and was batting around 600 in little league. I just came home from a game and as soon as I got in the door, my father asked me, "How many hits ya get, ya bastard?" He had his usual beer in hand and was in his typical semi-intoxicated state.

"Three!" I proudly replied.

"How many home runs?"

"None," I replied.

My introduction to training was when my father responded, "You weak son of a bitch. Get on the floor and do pushups."

I did only three, and he really tore into me for that. I usually managed to make a positive out of most of the negative childhood situations with my father. He made me do pushups every night before bed, and soon I began to love the exercise because I felt stronger, which in turn raised my confidence and self-esteem; and I began hitting some home runs. Soon I was doing 90 pushups in a row.

I put up a chinning bar in the basement and was up to 18 in no time. I made a wrist roller. I walked around constantly squeezing rubber balls to strengthen my wrists because that was what Ted

Williams did. I was hooked on training at an early age.

It was during this time that I bought my first copies of *Strength and Health* and *Muscular Development* magazines. I was buying baseball cards near a magazine rack and a cover caught my eye. *Muscular Development* was a new magazine at that time (1964), and John Grimek was the editor. From my first glance of him, I was in awe, but greatly inspired. I always read every word in *MD* and liked it even more than *S&H*, because of Grimek's influence. (I didn't even know about *Iron Man* 'til a few years later.)

I continued to lift cement blocks and copper tubing stored in the cellar, and did pushups, chins, dips between chairs, wrist roller work, situps and other calisthenics until I got my first York 110-pound barbell set for my birthday at age 13.

I was a fanatic and devoured everything related to training I could get my hands on. I was sad when I'd read all the articles in a new issue. I couldn't wait 'til the next month so I could ride my bike to the apothecary in Sherborn, Massachusetts, and buy the next issue.

I can remember the smell of the ink in the new issues. I had to hide the magazines because my father thought all the bodybuilders were "musclebound," but I knew better. My biggest heroes were Bob Hoffman and, especially, John Grimek. I still have a deep affection for and loyalty to the tradition of the York Barbell Company, and tremendous respect for its pivotal role, since the thirties, in the development of the Iron Game. To this day I will only buy York weights.

This background information is important because it should help you to understand the magnitude of the thrill I had in April 1976 when I drove to York, Pennsylvania, and met John Grimek. For an Iron Game/Physical Culture enthusiast, this was the equivalent of a baseball fan meeting Babe Ruth. I'd hoped to meet Bob Hoffman too.

I remember looking at all of Hoffman's medals and spending an hour or so in the museum section downstairs. I finally got the nerve up to ask if I could meet Bob Hoffman, but was told he was not in that day. I still regret not meeting him. But Grimek was upstairs in his office, and I was told that he would be happy to see me. My heart raced as I walked up a creaky staircase to his office. I sheepishly knocked on the office door and politely referred to him as Mr. Grimek.

Mr. Grimek invited me in and was extremely friendly. I was only 21 at the time and was completely in awe. At first I was surprised because he was well into his sixties at the time, but most of the photos I'd seen of him were not recent. He was in great shape, though, and I could tell that he still trained hard and regularly. He had his shirt sleeves rolled up, and I could see his huge biceps in full glory. He looked at least 20 years younger than most men of his age.

He asked me as many questions about my training, and my life in general, as I asked him. He seemed genuinely interested in me and I was impressed at how approachable and kind-hearted he was. He answered every question I had and was in no rush to have me leave. He signed an autograph for me that I guard with my life and proudly display on a wall of my gym. After asking every possible question I could think of, and spending about 30 minutes in his office, I felt I might start to be a pest. I thanked Mr. Grimek for his time, shook his hand, and let him get back to his work.

Dispelling Myths

It wasn't until fairly recently that the term "musclebound" has finally been put to rest. You may hear it once in a while now, but mainly by ignorant people. Most people today believe that strength training is beneficial. It wasn't always that way, and as a kid growing up I would always hear about it and be discouraged from lifting. I never believed it was true, mainly because of the hard work and courage of John Grimek and Bob Hoffman, who told me the truth.

On April 4, 1940 Bob Hoffman brought several members of the York Barbell Club, including John Grimek, to Springfield College. Dr. Karpovich, of Springfield College, had been influential in pushing "musclebound" theories throughout academia, and was making most athletic coaches shy away from training with weights. Strength training was being seriously threatened, and John Grimek was instrumental in turning this around. After Grimek was introduced to the panel, the pompous academics sneered at him and seemed to mock him at first, believing he was nothing but a big clumsy oaf with limited movement and "bound" muscles.

Grimek went right up to each of them and said, "Can you do this?" He then proceeded to contort his body into every stretch and bend possible, and reportedly could come close to touching his elbows to the floor while keeping his knees straight! Each of the academics gave a pitiful performance of flexibility when responding to the challenge, to which Grimek replied, something to the effect of, "You're musclebound, not me!"

Hoffman then had Grimek and others perform all kinds of feats including one-arm chins, handstands, backbends, jumping splits and numerous stretches. After Karpovich had witnessed this, he was stunned. By the time Hoffman and Grimek got through with Karpovich, he changed his position to, "There's no such thing as musclebound."

Hoffman went further and challenged any athlete in any sport to compete against his York Barbell Club in any physical test outside of their own specific sport. The challenge was widely publicized. There were no takers, mostly because of the larger-than-life image of Grimek and the fear that he would humiliate any challenger.

Our Responsibility

John Grimek was larger than life, much like John Wayne was. John was what the Iron Game and Physical Culture are really all about. He was the essence of how things were and how things should still be. When you think of John Grimek, you think of the glory days of the Iron Game before drugs ruined the honest competition, and the brotherhood.

The "good guys" in the Iron Game today have a sacred duty to carry on the tradition that John Grimek stood for and which Vic Boff and others still represent. Give no respect to steroid users— they are scum. Take down their pictures. Always keep your focus on good health as the primary motivation for your toil, and build muscle the old fashioned away—earn it by hard work and dedication, like John Grimek did.

THE NOBLE
HERITAGE...PHYSICAL
CULTURE

May 1999

The key to building natural strength is dedicated effort, and not just in the gym. Although there are surely vast differences in individual genetics, I know of no one who has not made tremendous gains over the long haul if they truly paid their dues. Many people "micro-manage" their training and worry overly about minor things, but somehow overlook the main issue—consistent dedication. Many assume that they are dedicated when, in fact, they are not. Some assume that they are dedicated just because they avidly read about strength training. But if you were to ask them what they ate yesterday, or how much sleep they got, or how they are actually progressing in their training, you'll frequently receive only excuses.

Dedication in natural strength training is best defined by the old-time term "Physical Culture." You don't hear this term too often anymore because it encompasses a way of life. It's not an end result, a trophy or a bodypart measurement, but a total lifestyle commitment. It's about how you live your life "in the dark" when no one is watching you. It's dedication to a 24-hour day philosophy, not just what you do in the gym. Most of the old-timers had this Physical Culture philosophy. They cared about health as much as strength. Just look at the old magazine titles. Today, it seems to me that most strong men couldn't care less about health. Steroid use is rampant, and you'll find many strong men smoking cigarettes and using recreational drugs too. They are no more dedicated to health than the average citizen.

Vic Boff is a good friend of mine, and we sometimes burn up the phone lines for hours. He's a wealth of knowledge and has endless stories about the old-timers. He personally knew many of them, and was very close with Sig Klein and George Jowett. No one hates steroids more than Vic Boff; and no one hates more than he does what has happened to the Iron Game as a result of steroids.

To build muscle naturally you have to do the hard exercises, be mentally tough, get enough sleep, eat the right foods and avoid the wrong foods, and sweat buckets for years and years. It takes dedication to do it the right way. You have to love it to be able to stick with it for decades; but the long-term rewards make it all worthwhile.

Building muscle on "tuna and baked potatoes" is a lot slower than building it on steroids. Undedicated phonies can build muscle fast on steroids, but they lose it fast and die young too. To me, a true champion lives a dedicated life of Physical Culture in the spirit of our founding fathers. Vic, for example, puts health first and has lived his life as a dedicated Physical Culture disciple. How many of today's "Mr. Something" drug-using bodybuilding "stars" will be the picture of health, strong, full of energy, and sharp as a tack like Vic when they get into their eighties? Not many, if any.

Almost every month I hear of another former bodybuilding star, or athlete, who is either dying from steroid use, or who recently died prematurely. And yet these are the guys that many of the ignorant and misinformed masses have looked to for training advice. Thank God for *Hardgainer* and the few other good training magazines that provide truthful information for drug-free trainees.

We have much more information today about health than our forefathers had, and we should be held to higher standards because of it. Some of the old-timers had bad habits, but overall they were dedicated to health based on the information they had available at the time. Most of the (few) unhealthy things they did were done unknowingly. Today there's no excuse.

I give a two hour Physical Culture orientation to all my regular clients (who are not just visitors), and this is done before any weights are lifted. I stress dedication, commitment to health, as well as strength. I've put the basic framework of the orientation into a tongue-in-cheek "Ten Commandments" format—the "Whelan Strength Training Commandments."

Whelan Strength Training Commandments

1. Thou shalt train for strength, whole-body fitness and health; and do cardiovascular exercise and flexibility training as well as strength training.

2. Thou shalt not smoke, take illegal drugs or abuse legal drugs.

3. Thou shalt not use steroids or assist anyone in obtaining them.

4. Thou shalt be mentally focused and give 100% effort at every training session.

5. Thou shalt strive for progressive resistance, using good form, without excessive rest between sets, and use the fullest (but safe) range of motion possible.

6. Thou shalt primarily focus on the basic compound strength training movements—multi-joint, not isolation—and train the whole body with equal emphasis on pushing and pulling. The training foundation is overhead pushing/ pulling, horizontal pushing/pulling, and leg, hip and back pushing/pulling.

7. Thou shalt not seek shortcuts, miracle formulas or gimmicks, but instead stick to basic and sound information concerning training and nutrition, such as *Hardgainer, Brawn, Beyond Brawn* and *The Insider's Tell-All Handbook on Weight-Training Technique.*

8. Thou shalt perform hard progressive strength training, and not toning, shaping, or bodysculpting.

133

9. Thou shalt not train "bodyparts" but train the whole body (hard) usually about twice every 7-10 days.

10. Thou shalt not rely on mega-hype muscle mags for training or nutritional advice.

All of my clients get a copy of this, and even though it's in a humorous format, the rules are taken very seriously. I have, for example, expelled people from my facility who lied when they told me that they were non-smokers. I don't want these types, and usually get rid of them over the phone. I have had many requests for the "WST Commandments," and so have included them in this article.

Bodyparts Training and Natural Training Don't Mix

Most people who train "bodyparts" (not the whole body) confuse "training" with "going to the gym." They somehow believe that by going into a building called "the gym" they will get bigger and stronger. They rarely talk about intensity or how hard they worked, but instead talk about being in a building. They brag about how long they are "in the gym," and how often they "go to the gym." They believe that by training "bodyparts," and thus spending more time "in the gym," they will get better results. They are usually unsophisticated beginners who feel more advanced just because they train in a bodyparts format. They don't realize that bodyparts training has been around for decades and is nothing new.

Guys who "go to the gym" usually spend more time talking (about sports and politics, for example), and socializing at the water fountain, than they do training. That's why they are there for three hours! They take a ten-minute rest between sets, and usually bench press with several other people. Their bench press workout alone takes 45 minutes. These guys rarely even break a sweat!

It's almost impossible to train bodyparts without overtraining from "muscle overlap." You can't put the major multi-joint exercises into neat, separate categories. The bench press, for example, does not hit just the chest, but front delts and triceps. The machine pullover, termed the "upper-body squat" by Arthur Jones, works almost every muscle in the upper body. What category do you put it in? The truth is that if you train bodyparts 5-6 days per week, you're either on drugs or are not working hard—you take long rests between sets, and your workout is filled with easy exercises such as triceps kickbacks, cable crossovers, lateral raises, flyes, leg extensions, etc.; and you don't do squats, deadlifts, chins, rows, military presses, etc.

If you train *hard*, and are natural, you *can't* train bodyparts 5-6 days per week. If you train hard, whole body, you'll be physically unable to train more than twice every 7-10 days. Anyone who does not believe this can come for a free workout. It would be my pleasure to "convince" him.

"Look of Power"

Dr. Ken and others have written articles about "the look of power." You don't get the look of power unless you do the heavy compound exercises—the ones which require lots of recovery time for natural guys. Dr. Ken described this well when he stated that people who do bodyparts training look like they are just a "collection of bodyparts" that don't seem to fit together. When you have the look of power you're thick and look strong from *any* angle. Even if you have a raincoat on you *still* look thick and strong.

The look of power means thickness in the back, traps, glutes, legs, neck and whole body, not just arms and chest. If people only know that you "lift weights" when you have a tank top on, you don't have the look of power. The look of power can't be hidden. It has nothing to do with cuts or definition, but size and thickness. If you have the look of power, then no matter what oversize baggy sweatshirt you have on, you'll still look powerful.

It's no accident that bodyparts training and drug use grew together

135

and are from the same roots. Most people get innocently sucked into bodyparts training without realizing it. The truth is that "bodyparts routines" are usually "drug routines" (or "wimp routines") and are not effective for the average drug-free trainee.

I love to get "bodyparts types" to train with me, especially if they have a cocky attitude. If they say things like, "Are you sure that twice a week will be enough?" I go out of my way to change their thinking.

To do this, I'll have them spend the first workout doing heavy high-rep leg work for twenty minutes—and they usually don't last even that long. If they do, I keep them going with little rest between sets doing nothing but the hard stuff, to failure; and they finish with the sandbag carry (if they last that long). This is strictly an attitude-adjustment workout, and is only used for "special" people.

When people come in with a really good attitude, and listen, then I start them much slower and pick up the intensity over a period of time, to build up conditioning progressively.

The smart ass types usually last only about twenty minutes of an attitude-adjustment workout, and are then laying on the floor. They are usually amazed at how soaked in sweat they are, and how tired. I then love to ask them, "Do you think we hit your biceps and back enough? Why don't you come back tomorrow?" They never do, and are usually too sore and tired to think about training for at least three or four days, the way it should be.

"COMMON SENSE"
PERIODIZATION

July 1999

Periodization means "to divide into periods," when defined by most dictionaries. That's also the way that I view this term as it applies to strength training. I'm a big believer that some form of change in a routine every three or four months or so is as good mentally as it is physically. In addition to this, as noted in some previous articles, I like to have a day or two each month when I mix things up a little bit. The change keeps enthusiasm high, helps you through sticking points, bolsters your motivation, and re-energizes your training.

I want to be very clear on one thing. When I use the word "periodization"—I actually call it "common sense periodization"—I'm not advocating the orthodox definition used by the NSCA and some other organizations. I find that definition illogical. I don't believe in a "hypertrophy phase" as being separate from a "strength-building" phase. There are also other aspects of the orthodox definition that I don't agree with, but rather than get into all of that I'd rather just focus on my definition.

If you love strength training, as I do, then "common sense" periodization is great. You can try many training methods and find what works best for you, or just what you enjoy best. You may find that several methods work well for you, as I have. Personally, I look forward to the change after about every four months. Even though many strength-training methods absolutely do work, at least for some people, what determines what works *for you* is often in your head—it's the "enjoyment factor." This factor should be strongly considered when you choose a training mode or method. You should enjoy training. You will not stick with something, or do well at it, if you dislike it. Find a method that you like. There are many schools of thought in this field, and several of them are good. The problem is that many people, especially beginners, get confused and need to label the type of training they do. Forget the labels. There are also many dogmatic writers and organizations who think you're scum unless you train exactly like they do. Ignore these people.

Many people label me as a "high-intensity training" (HIT) advocate; in fact, I've even used this description of myself, so I don't mind the label. But I also do many things that are not standard "party line" HIT. I spend a good part of the year doing lower reps. In some articles I've even coined my training as "lower-rep HIT." But this is just for part of the year. With my clients we still do the higher reps too, such as 20- and even 30-rep squats, fifties days, etc. I occasionally do singles (myself), but rarely with clients. The best way to describe my type of training is "natural, hard, safe and progressive."

An Illustration

I sometimes do multiple work sets, but never more than 3. In fact, I've spent most of my training life doing 3 work sets per exercise, but my friendship with Drew Israel influenced me to try one-set-to-failure (for work sets). For the last few years I've used the one-set-to-failure approach a lot, and experienced great results.

I'll be 45 this summer, and I'm at all-time personal best strength levels in most exercises. I recently got 360 for 9, followed by 390 for 5 and 410 for 3 on the Hammer Incline Press. (I usually do just one work set, but felt so strong that workout that I wanted to test myself.) About three years ago when I visited Drew in New York ("Training and Eating in The Big Apple," in issue #45), I barely got a single rep with 400 pounds, and that was a PR at the time. Additionally, I recently got 255 for 10 on the Nautilus Power Plus Military Press, 300 for 9 on the Hammer Iso Row and 555 for 12 on the Hammer Iso Leg Press. All PR's. I'm a lot stronger than I was a few years ago, and probably ever. Isn't this stuff great? In fact, one-set-to-failure training has helped me a lot.

138

If you ever use one-set-to-failure training you will burn fewer calories than you would with multiple-set work, so you must either make up for this by consuming fewer calories, or by doing more cardiovascular exercise. Keep this in mind if you notice your bodyfat creeping up when you switch to one-set training.

I still use 2 or 3 work sets for most of my clients on most exercises. I believe that one-set-to-failure works better for the older experienced trainee with a solid training foundation, who *truly* understands what it means to go to failure. Many newcomers don't understand this, have no training base, and end their sets 1 or 2 reps prematurely. You can experiment with your number of sets in the common sense periodization format. Do 2 or 3 work sets per exercise for four months, and then try just a single work set to failure per exercise for four months. Take good notes and trust your own instincts.

Machines or Free Weights?

I don't consider machines to be superior to free weights. I spent most of my training life using free weights almost exclusively but with any piece of equipment, it's how you use the device that counts. My use of some machines now is mainly a business decision. It makes my job a lot easier because I change plates and spot people all day. Machines also reduce my liability and the chance of injury for my older clients, some of whom have little experience when they start.

If you've access to both the *good* machines and free weights, common sense periodization is a way to enable you to use both. For example, do the Hammer Chest Press for four months then do free-weights incline presses for four months.

Free weights are not "more manly," and neither are machines "for wimps," as some people have written. Anyone who has used the Tru-Squat can attest to that. Machines and free weights are both good. Dr. Ken, Drew Israel, Dan Riley, Ken Mannie and others are huge machine advocates. Use what you like, and ignore the critics.

Odd-Object Lifting

Odd objects are also something to consider using to add variety. I don't do this type of training on a regular basis (at every training session) but as a change of pace every few weeks. My clients are usually hammered after the (regular equipment) workout, so the finishers would be like swatting a fly with a sledgehammer, and lead to overtraining if done on a regular basis. We will, for example, do the sandbag carry or farmer's walk as a "finisher" after all the barbell and machine work is done, but not to replace any of it.

I'm not an advocate of training exclusively with odd objects (to replace machines or barbells) for an entire periodization cycle, or even for just one entire workout. Everything old is not always good or better. A sandbag curl is not nearly as good as a barbell curl. You can't hold onto a sandbag well, and even though it may toughen your hands, it will not work your biceps as well because you can't hold onto enough weight. Don't make the mistake of sacrificing major muscle groups in the name of "grip work." It's usually better to do the grip work separately.

There are many modern devices that are a definite improvement over what they had 50 or 60 years ago. Do you think that John Grimek would have done free-style leg presses with weights balancing on his shoes, like in the old Mark Berry poster, if he could have used a Hammer Leg Press instead? C'mon now! John wasn't a fool.

Though odd object may be trendy in very limited circles, odd objects are inferior to a barbell or Hammer Strength/Southern Xercise type machines for use on an ongoing basis where progression is monitored. Additionally, if you're only training *yourself*, that's one thing, but when you're responsible for the well-being of others—who are entrusting you with their bodies—you must use a safer mode than anvils and barrels, etc. The sandbag carry or farmer's walk however, as a finisher for the young or well conditioned trainee (or athlete) is a fine addition to a workout.

Rep Speed

Even speed of motion can be experimented with. We use an 8-second rep speed workout once in a while as a change of pace, and it's brutal. Dick Conner does the same thing at The Pit. Dick notes, and I agree, "Slow training is definitely not for wimps. Anyone who says it is, has never tried it as I use it."

The problem I have with slow training is not the actual training, but the dogmatic individuals who represent this philosophy. Many in this camp also put no emphasis on progression, and are virtually nothing but glorified "toners." Slow training can be a great change of pace and even a permanent way to train if you like, as long as you make *progression* a top priority, as Drew Israel does.

Summary

Don't get caught up in the trends or the philosophical catfights. Many methods work. Life is too short, so enjoy your training and *experiment* (sensibly, of course). Consider changing your rep ranges, exercises and various modes and methods every four months or so, while sticking to the basic core philosophy. The only definition or label you need is "natural, hard, safe and progressive."

MENTAL ASPECTS OF STRENGTH TRAINING: PART I

September 1999

I gave a presentation at Matt Brzycki's clinic at Princeton University about the mental aspects of training, and it was well received. I covered the topic from two angles: the trainee's perspective, and the coach's. The latter in particular is very neglected, and really needs to be addressed.

There have been many articles written on the mental aspects of training, but few have covered the mental aspects of coaching. I'm going to start with a different take here, and begin with the mental aspects of coaching. I'll cover the mental aspects of training from the trainee's point of view in the next issue. I've had so many people ask "How do you do things?" This article is basically my coaching philosophy from a mental standpoint.

The Priority

First and foremost, to be a good strength coach you must have your trainees' best interests at heart. The primary goal of a good coach is to get each trainee through the planned workout. It's easy to drop someone; it's harder, and takes more effort and skill as a coach, to get your trainee through the planned workout. The whole body should be worked with balanced pushing and pulling, over the training week or workout, depending on recovery ability. If you clock your guy after just a few exercises, and he does not finish, he has an incomplete training program, which means incomplete progress and development.

The human body can only take so much, and anyone, no matter how good shape they are in, can easily be dropped. To deliberately plan to drop someone is lazy coaching. The only time that I'll do this, and think it's justified, is if there's a respect issue going on. If someone comes in with a know-it-all cocky attitude, and is not really listening to what I tell him, then I'll deliberately train him to drop him, but only if he's young and there's no fear of death. (Deaths are not good for business!) If they are older, I'll just ask them to leave. But as long as someone comes in with respect and trust, and listens—which the vast majority of people do—then it's my responsibility to do my best to get them through the planned workout. Good coaching is positive, not abusive. For beginners I usually expect about three weeks of training before they can complete my planned workout.

Of course, now and then someone may vomit due to an all-out effort, but this should never be the goal. The only reason I have a bucket is to avoid having a mess should vomiting happen. I don't like to have to use the bucket, but it's there when needed. Some people are prone to it, such as Vern Veldekens, who must have used it fifty times over the course of two years of training. Many others have never used the bucket. The bucket now has "Vern" on it, and was named in his honor when he left to go to medical school a year or so ago.

There are some coaches who don't think you've had a good workout unless you use the bucket. This is wrong. I view the bucket as getting a "purple heart" medal. You get a purple heart when you get wounded, but you don't want to get wounded. When you use the bucket, you get an "atta boy" for a good effort. *But it's never the goal.* A good workout is defined by more reps per set, or heavier weight used, or good effort, and is not defined by puking. Some of my strongest clients have *never* puked due to training.

A good coach must be a good judge of effort. Not everyone can give the same amount of effort. There are huge differences in ability. Nonetheless, whatever they can give, I want it all. You must be smart enough to recognize the differences in individuals, and be a good judge of effort. You must watch closely—see their expression and read them. Extracting effort is an art form. I try to push someone to the edge of the cliff, and just when he's about to fall off it, I pull him back. This is actually harder training because the trainee will still do *all* the planned work. Otherwise he would have just gone down and be KOed (whether he really is or isn't), and not finish the work.

I've seen many people, who are used to the quick KOed training philosophy, "take a dive" to get out of finishing the workout. It's easier to go down and act like you're all messed up than to actually finish the work. They are surprised when I give them a four minute rest and then continue and make them finish the rest of the workout.

Sometimes, extra rest is important at the right time, and helps complete the planned workout, which is of critical importance. It's my opinion that it's better to decrease intensity—i.e., give more rest at strategic workout points—in order to finish the planned work, than to have intensity so high for the whole workout that the trainee gets KOed early and can't finish. Until overall condition is built up, it's better to focus on finishing the work. Conditioning will catch up eventually, but at least the whole body would be receiving balanced training. To me it's an art form of manipulating exercise sequence to keep the trainee moving, but with easy exercises following the hardest ones, to give built-in recovery while not actually resting—my clients pay for an hour workout maximum, and have to finish in that time. For example, I would work the neck after the Tru Squat.

We usually go a whole hour, and it's brutal. At the beginning of the workout there's usually little rest, but near the end there will be a little more to enable the client to finish all the planned work.

Passion

I love strength training, and I love coaching other people to train. It's a labor of love. I feel so fortunate to be able to make a good living doing something that I absolutely love to do. I love going to work and getting up at 5 am. I can't wait to get started! I'm almost always enthusiastic! It's fun, rewarding, and as far as I'm concerned, the best job in the world.

144

To be good as a coach, you must have the passion for it! You can't just go through the motions, or else your clients will also go through the motions. I've learned over the years that almost everything in life flows from passion. Whatever you can think of, from business, to money, to clients, success *flows from passion*. You don't get into something for security. You make your own security. If you're a good artist and have the talent and passion, then you'll sell your art. You don't get into something just because of the money. God knows there are many stressed out and miserable lawyers. You can't fake passion. You either have it, or you don't. If you've got it, it makes your job a lot easier, and a lot more fun.

I try to instill this positive attitude, enthusiasm and love of training into my clients. Washington, DC, is a transient area. I want my clients totally "in the family," so if they transfer out of the area, they still stay "in the family" and are not sucked back onto the BS way of training ever again. I actually subsidize my clients to read good magazines. I let them deduct costs from what they pay me. Clients who learn about training, are interested in it, and enjoy it, will almost always be more successful.

Motivation

When you run a private operation, like I do at Whelan Strength Training, you sometimes have an advantage over a public institution or athletic teams. I can control the type of clients I want, as I have a strong training philosophy, and clients are paying to train with me. They have to be motivated and want to do this, or they would not be here. I also make them pre-pay for their workouts, so if they are lying in bed at 5 am, they will think twice about blowing me off—because they will lose their money. I could not do this in a small town out in the boondocks because there would not be enough people there for me to make a living from. Living in a large city enables me to have a strict training philosophy and stick with it. I only need about thirty crazy people in a city the size of Washington!

145

My clients must buy into the WST philosophy, or train somewhere else. Morale is much higher with strong leadership than it is with a weak training philosophy where anything goes, "as long as I get paid," which is how most so-called "personal trainers" operate. I refer to these types of trainers—with no backbone or solid philosophy—as "fitness prostitutes." They make the rest of us look bad.

Supervision

I like to refer to myself as a coach only because a coach has a philosophy. A coach does not ask you what you want to do, he tells you what you *need* to do. Supervision is also important as you're actively involved in the workout. You don't just write out workout cards and then daydream your way through the training sessions, like some coaches do. You must go through the workouts with the clients. You must motivate and supervise.

Coaching for a team or school is sometimes harder than in a private operation, because some of the athletes hate lifting weights and are only doing it because they have to. You must convince them that training is a "means to an end" and bind them to the benefit of training. You must "sell" training to them. You also need a head coach who totally supports the strength and conditioning program, and enforces strict attendance to workouts, etc. A program that recognizes and rewards those who train hard and have good attendance, and punishes those who slack off and have poor attendance, will usually be a solid and successful program.

Variety is good, but not too much. It's good to have somewhat of a pattern to your program. This enables your athletes to mentally prepare and visualize the training before the workout. Certain traditions that I have like a fifties day, sandbag day, etc., build morale. The athlete looks forward to the variety, and it's a good mental and physical change of pace.

As a coach, be prepared. Keep records, plan workouts ahead, organize ahead of time, and don't be fumbling and bumbling around. Know your people as individuals, and learn what makes them tick. There are different ways to motivate each one. Some respond well to pressure, but some don't. Some need a kick in the ass, while some never do. Keep good records and don't be afraid to lead. As a coach you must truly believe in your program or philosophy, or else your people never will. They will see right through you. Do what you believe in, and stick to your guns. This gives you the passion to lead.

MENTAL ASPECTS OF STRENGTH TRAINING: PART II

November 1999

In this issue I'm going to cover the mental aspects of training *from the lifter's perspective*. First and foremost, you have to *want* to train, otherwise no mental training will help you If you don't really like to train, then maybe you need to evaluate why you're training in the first place, and perhaps look for a new hobby—one that you really enjoy. I feel strongly that you should enjoy training.

Once you decide that you really want to do this, then you must realize how important the mind and proper thinking are to one's strength-training success. Before *every* workout you must clear your head of all outside thoughts and distractions. Whatever problems you may have, you must learn to leave them aside, and put them on the back burner. Everyone has problems—the only people who don't have problems are dead. The difference between successful and unsuccessful people is that successful people learn to manage their problems. Concentrate on what you're doing. Be here now! Before doing a set, take about 20 seconds to think of what you're about to do. Don't talk. If you were talking between sets, you must stop talking and focus on the task at hand for at least 20 seconds before lifting, or your set is doomed.

I took a graduate course in sports psychology under one of the best sports psychologist in the business—Bob Rotella, at the University of Virginia. One of the most helpful things I learned was that there are two main types of concentration. There's *narrow/internal* and *broad/external* concentration. External concentration is the type that's used by actors and performers on a stage. Usually outside cues are given by a director or conductor, etc. Peripheral signals, timing, and non-verbal communication by other actors, for example, must be noticed by a broad view or an outward concentration. This is exactly the sort of concentration you use

148

when gazing into a mirror. The problem is that this is the exact opposite of the type of concentration you need when you train! If you feel that you absolutely must use mirrors to learn technique, then use a bar with light weight to practice form, but this should not be considered actual training.

The argument that mirrors help your form is ridiculous, in my view! Most mirrors in gyms are not full length anyways, so you don't even see your lower body. Plus, you don't have eyes behind your head, so the muscles of the rear delts, hamstrings and most of your back, calves, triceps and glutes can't be seen. Are mirrors on the ceiling for the bench press? If people can do reverse slam dunks, and all sorts of other difficult moves like flips in gymnastics, and acrobatic stunts, without mirrors, then mirrors are surely not needed for simple things like curls.

The strongest people in the world—Olympic lifters, powerlifters and highland games athletes—don't use mirrors because they are in narrow, internal mode. If you're a strength coach at a gym with mirrors already in place, a good trick is to turn the heat way down, or the air conditioning way up, so that the guys will wear their long-sleeved shirts to keep warm. When covered up they won't be as likely to look at themselves in mirrors, and will keep their thinking functional.

Narrow, internal concentration is the type used when strength training. Your mind is focused on the task at hand like a laser beam, and nothing but the task at hand exists in your mind. A bomb could go off and if you were in a good narrow/internal state, you would not even hear it, because your mind would be connected exclusively to the objective and nothing else.

I try to instill in all my clients the importance of building an *attitude foundation*, and not just in the weight room, but for life as a whole. As I've noted in earlier articles, I've a reading list of positive thinking books and motivational cassette tapes that I recommend my clients to buy. Any books by Zig Ziglar, Norman Vincent Peale, Og Mandino, David Schwartz or Robert Schuller are strongly recommended. My favorite motivational book is *The Magic of Thinking Big,* by David Schwartz. I've read that book at least twenty times. When you build an attitude foundation, you take control of your life and eliminate excuses from your vocabulary. Anyone can have a good attitude when things are going well, *but a champion has a good attitude when things are going badly.* This means that things should turn around and start going well again soon. When you think positively, you see opportunity in almost every situation, and always learn to see the good in things. When you're in a negative state of mind, you miss most opportunities. You must also eliminate the word "luck" from your vocabulary. Luck is when opportunity and determination meet.

Anger as a Positive Force

When strength training, it's very helpful to get angry. You must attack the weights as if they were going to attack your family. You're going to war with the weights. It's not only a matter of positive thinking—you must combine anger with the positive thinking. If you saw the movie "The Water Boy," it gave some extreme and even hilarious examples of channeling anger in a positive way, and illustrates what I mean. Channel your frustrations into the exercise. Not only will you be stronger, you'll reduce your stress level and be more relaxed later. *Channel anger or frustration towards the exercise, not towards yourself.* Give it your best effort and then move to the next exercise. Don't sulk or whine if you did not hit the goal. Just do your best and then drop it! Otherwise your next set will be affected. Remember that Babe

Ruth struck out 1,330 times and hit 714 home runs. The strange thing is that no one even remembers the strike outs. The thing to remember is that The Babe kept swinging the bat. If you keep giving honest effort, you'll get your dues in terms of poundage increases.

Think of yourself as big and strong (even if you're not yet); use power thinking not weak thinking. You are what you think about, and will be dictated by your most dominant thoughts. Don't think of yourself as being genetically disadvantaged, etc. Don't limit yourself. Have *realistically* high expectations. Aim high. Have goals. You can't hit a target if you don't have one. Write down your goals, and dwell on them. I repeat—*write them down.* One of the biggest traits of underachievers is that they never put their goals on paper. Believe you'll achieve your goals, and most likely you will. Remember the Henry Ford quote: "Whether you think you can or think you can't, you're right!" That sums it up well. Much has been written about the power of belief. Just as a prayer without belief is worthless, and an insult to God, any mental techniques without true belief are also worthless.

Visualize good hard workouts. Complete many workouts in your head. Never miss lifts in your mind. Try to have time each day to go over the planned workout in your head. Dream creatively and see yourself breaking new personal records—feel them, see them and smell them. See yourself as a winner, respected and a champion. Know the difference between confidence and arrogance. Being confident and feeling good about yourself is a good thing, but treat others with respect. Don't look up or down at anyone, but straight in the eye.

The most important language you have is the one you use to talk to yourself. What you say to yourself, and what you believe about yourself, can have miraculous as well as devastating effects. What you say, think and believe about yourself affects not only your cognitive thinking, but also your subconscious mind. Your subconscious mind is extremely powerful and is essentially your emotional personality. Never use negative language to yourself.
When Tony Gwynn strikes out, he does not say, "I suck," or "I can't hit." He says "I was not at my best today, but expect to be ready tomorrow." This is a good example of positive self talk. Always, and especially *during* workouts, use positive self talk. Your subconscious mind is much larger than your conscious/thinking mind. You can't say negative things about yourself without getting hurt.

Sometimes it's good to learn to take the pressure off! This was especially important to me during my powerlifting competitions. I would attack the weights with abandon because I would tell myself, "What's the worst thing that could happen? I just miss the lift! So what? I'm not going to die or anything!" This took the pressure off at critical times, and helped a great deal. Another pressure-reducing technique is to always think of only competing against yourself, and not others. If you compete against yourself, you always win. You can't lose when you compete against yourself.

Finally, learn instinctive, confidence-building tricks. Timely changes in goals when in a rut can work wonders. Sometimes, adding weight when in a rut helps because you have a built-in excuse, and no pressure. You know it's your best weight ever, so past failures are erased from your mind. As I've reported in an earlier article, back in 1975 I was stuck for months at a maximum bench press of 295 pounds. Three hundred was a major psych job for me. I finally increased the weight to 305 and had no pressure or past failures in my mind. The weight flew up with no problem the first time I tried it.

Give top priority to the mental aspects of your life, not just in your training, but for everything. It will greatly help your training for sure, but so much more than that too.

DEDICATION & DOING

January 2000

Use the Best Tool Available

I'm an Iron Game guy. I study the old books and magazines and love reading about the old-timers. My training philosophy is a combination of the best information from the old-timers mixed with the best modern information. I was raised exclusively on free weights, but now use a lot of the good quality plate-loaded machines too. I didn't just collect machines like some people do, and I don't really enjoy talking about them. I just use them. I care more about the strength of the person using the machine, than the strength curve of the machine. I don't believe that, overall, barbells are better, or machines are better. They both work. I believe that you should use the best tool you have available.

If you're lucky enough to have some of the great new machines, then by all means use them. But if you don't have them, don't fret. You still have enough to get the job done, and done well too.

There are many people who have an opposite view, and can be described as machine snobs. They have no idea who George Jowett was, and would rather talk about the latest Med-Ex machine, but not how much they lifted on it, just the machine itself! Many of these types would rather polish their machine than use it. They constantly buy the newest machines and talk more about the machines they have than their actual training. They believe that training is inferior on anything less than the latest or newest machine. Once you get a few machines, you can get into, and distracted by, a whole new machine network. It's amazing.

I never had any machines until about four years ago. For many years I trained only with York bars and plates, and Jubinville gear. Just for me, this stuff was great; but when I train ten people in a row, I can get exhausted because my job becomes more that of a laborer, little different from a bricklayer because of all the plate changing and moving around of equipment. The Hammer Strength and Southern Xercise machines I now have are great, and make my job a lot easier. I love using them.

A lot of guys call me and almost apologize for not having a certain machine, and use this as an excuse for poor training. My philosophy about the good plate-loaded machines is that they are nothing more than "guided barbells"—just alternative tools to get the job done. But they should be viewed as secondary to the work being done, not the main reason for training success.

I had some of the best workouts of my life in crude, poorly equipped gyms. It's passion, effort, desire and consistent hard work that makes just a simple barbell work wonders. You don't really need anything more. At a small, dingy, minimally equipped gym at Bitburg Airbase in Germany, from 1976-1979, I had some of the best workouts of my life. The showers frequently had only cold water. The cables on the pulley machines were always broken. Someone was always painting something for an inspection. (In the military, anything that doesn't move gets painted.)

Even the barbell plates were painted several times during this period. They were black, gold, and white at different times. A few times they were still wet when we came to train, as someone had painted them in the middle of the day. We still lifted and got paint all over us. As long as there were bars and plates, we were happy!

Doing, Not Talking—Just Lift!

Respect is earned by doing, but it's not just how much you lift that earns respect. It's about effort. Those who are willing to put forth effort and dedication are the ones that earn respect and promote camaraderie and brotherhood. It's hard not to like a guy who works his ass off! It's hard not to respect a coach who works your ass off. Even a beginner who is not strong will be respected and liked if he works hard. People who train hard themselves usually respect others who train hard. They respect hard work because they do it too. They know how it feels. They understand how tough it is. It's frequently the person who doesn't train hard himself, that loves to foster division and ill will, and argue about minor training issues.

On average, the guys who are successful in strength training love to train. They don't miss workouts. They find a way to train. They don't make excuses why they can't train. They make do with the equipment they have available, not complain about which new machine they don't have. They don't just talk about training, read about it, write on the internet about it, or make excuses about why they can't do it. Instead, they lift—hard and regularly. These people are the backbone of the Iron Game. They are the passion and beauty of modern strength training. These guys are my brothers—people who work hard, sweat buckets, and move great poundages regularly and diligently in the icy cold garages of New England, in the barns of Iowa, or in the basements of London.

These are regular people who train with a tenacity and dedication that is anything but regular. They do this because they love it. They believe in it. It's almost spiritual to them. They get no money, fame or glory for it. No one is making them do it; they just do it for themselves. They love getting stronger but would never dream of taking steroids to gain strength. They just love to train hard and stretch their natural physical capacity to the limit. They live their lives by the sacred code of our physical culture forefathers.

You earn respect only by doing—not by talking. Nothing turns me off more than a so-called expert who doesn't even train. But there are many of them. Many conferences and seminars are given by guys with 12-inch necks! It's incredible. These are the type of people who sometimes spend hours each day on the internet arguing about strength training philosophy. They love to attack or put down others, and hide behind a computer screen, usually thousands of miles away. Many of the Ph.D. researcher types fall into this category. They can talk forever about the human physiological response to strength training. However, they know nothing about real-world strength training because they don't do it themselves.

Brotherhood of Iron

I'm talking about guys like my friend Jon Schultheis of Keansburg,

New Jersey. Jon is one of the strongest and most dedicated natural guys around. He has come down to train at WST several times, and I've put him through some brutal workouts. He loves to train hard and always comes back for more. Jim Duggan of Seaford, New York, is another good example of dedication and hard work. Jim does not talk much, but boy does he lift! He is a lifetime natural lifter and can bench press over 400 pounds for several reps with a three-inch bar! Jim is one of the best natural lifters of all time.

There are many more people like them, and I wish I could mention them all. They all deserve recognition, and define what strength training is all about—the pure love of training, *the camaraderie of effort.*

We share this common goal and common bond that unites us—passion for natural strength and hard training, i.e., the brotherhood of iron, strength and hard work. All are welcome if they are willing to pay the price. Race, religion, politics or nationality don't matter when you're battling iron. Citizenship to this nation requires only effort and doing, not excuses and theorizing.

Dedication and Gym Atmosphere

My best training partner ever was Glenn Pieschke. We trained together at the poorly equipped gym at Bitburg Airbase in Germany. We trained like we owned the place. Whenever we went for a personal record, we would let everyone know about it. We would run all around the gym and tell everyone—on the racquetball courts, basketball court, everywhere. Anyone who was interested, and there were many, would be brought to the weight room. Some thought we were crazy, but wanted to see what all the fuss was about.

We loved to put friendly pressure on each other. The whole gym would root us on. I remember when I benched 350 for the first time, Glenn had organized a large crowd. After completing the lift, I yelled, "350 pounds! Enough weight to crush the average human being! Go home and tell your mothers!" We were cocky, but friendly. People loved it. It got them psyched! Soon, every guy in the weight room was doing the same thing.

We rooted for each other. There was a lot of back slapping, screaming, yelling, grunting, groaning and sweating. We had a sort of "gang," and if someone wasn't there, we all knew it and would get on his case when we saw him at the chow hall. There was peer pressure to train. The weight room was dark, damp and cold; but to us, it was warm, bright, and full of energy and life. We loved that place! Weights were banging everywhere, and 10s, 5s and 2-1/2s were tossed back and forth around the room. Everyone had chalk; in fact, it was all over us! We had a true brotherhood, and so much fun training.

We would train come sleet or snow. Even base alerts (war games) didn't stop us. We usually worked 24-hour shifts, but when your shift was over, you had free time. But you still had to comply with the "war" conditions if you remained on the base. Most guys would get the hell out of Dodge after they ate and slept. We would bring our gas masks to the gym and still train. I can remember squatting in my gas mask. That was real high-intensity training!

Glenn broke his lower leg (tibia), but kept training while it healed, and even squatted with his cast on. He put a ten-pound plate under the shoe of his good leg to offset the heel bump on his cast. We never missed a workout, grew like crazy, and made tremendous progress. Anyone who trained with us at Bitburg would have made at least as much progress as they ever had anywhere else. That we only had very basic equipment just didn't matter.

ARCH ENEMIES OF PHYSICAL CULTURE

March 2000

The first thing I do when talking to new clients is have them burn any of the modern mega-hype muscle magazines that they own (and to never read them in the future). As readers should know, those magazines glorify drug-using bodybuilders and try to portray them as the picture of health, strength and hard work when nothing could be further from the truth. There are lies, cheap gimmicks and worthless advice on almost every page. About half the magazines' content is taken up with huge ads of "miracle" supplements and "magic" potions.

How many of these ads do you see in *Hardgainer*? None! Stuart is more interested in getting out the truth than earning money. The mega-hype mags are not. Those publications are far less truthful than even the tabloid newspapers at the checkout stand. They cleverly combine a micro element of truth with about 95% bull, a lot of pictures, sex and hype to sell this crap to millions. It's sad and incredible to think that many individuals actually believe it! At least with the tabloid papers, most people read them for fun but don't really believe what they read. The mega-hype mags are so harmful and dangerous because they pass themselves off as truthful. They are truly the worst of a group I've coined as "The Fitness Prostitutes."

The ads they use are a joke. I can't believe how so many people get suckered into them. They work something like this: You find a guy who is already big, like an advanced, seasoned drug-using bodybuilder. Have him stop training (and stop taking steroids too), and just eat ice cream and junk food for about four months. Then, you do the photo shoot for the before picture, but you make sure that the guy has a hangover, does not smile, has no tan, has not combed his hair or even shaven, wears glasses, and sticks out his gut as far as possible. Have him hold up a newspaper to "prove"

158

the date. Now, for the next three months, the guy goes back to his previous training, but trains harder than ever, with an hour of cardio almost every day too. He goes on a strict diet, takes a ton of steroids, and also makes sure to get a good tan. On the day of the after photo, he gets a haircut, shaves and wears contacts. Then for the actual shot he sucks in his gut and smiles. And I almost forgot, he took the "magic" supplement every day of the three months prior to the *after* photo!

There's also a lot of phony information (propaganda) being put out by various sports/bodybuilding organizations about conformity with drug testing and a sudden ability of testing to keep the sport clean. Bull! Bull! Bull! Nothing could be more false. They would have you believe that the performance-enhancing drug problem is a thing of the past, and that drug testing is now keeping things clean and under control. Many of the bodybuilding and various lifting organizations want you to believe this; but the truth is that they couldn't care less about the drug problem. They only care about the public *perception* of it. There's no bigger offender than the sport of bodybuilding.

Bodybuilding as it is today is a disgrace. As long as the organizations that run modern bodybuilding can pimp the big drug-using stars to push worthless supplements down your throat, they are happy. The old Physical Culture values of health, honest effort, and the reward for living a disciplined life, is gone. The Physical Culture camaraderie of hard training, health and integrity was a part of John-Grimek-type of bodybuilding. It has no place in today's bodybuilding. Truthful information is of no concern for the leaders of today's bodybuilding.

Please don't be fooled by the phony statistics that claim drug testing to be effective. Drug use by athletes—especially bodybuilders, powerlifters and other strength athletes—is higher than ever right now. The users are just not getting caught. There are now hundreds of drugs to improve sports performance. Many of them can't even be detected because a test for them has yet to be developed. Even many of the drugs that can be tested for can be altered with "masking agents," so the user will usually still test clean even though he's on the stuff. The technology for beating drug tests and getting athletes to test clean is far ahead of the advances to catch the cheaters.

There are many crooked doctors, chemists and self-trained (ex-bodybuilder type) steroid experts who get paid big bucks from bodybuilders, lifters and all types of world-class athletes to help them use drugs and get away with it. They are known as "drug gurus." They mix and develop custom "designer-type" steroids that are "stealth-like" and undetectable due to the masking agent that has altered the original drug. They also have drugs for which there's currently no test developed, such as human growth hormone, which is probably the most commonly used banned substance by elite athletes today, despite the fact that it's extremely expensive.

Most tests for anabolic steroids only work conclusively on pure, unaltered, commercially available steroids. Most of today's users are sophisticated enough to know this, and do not get caught because of it. They know that the tester is looking for a very specific result for each drug tested for. When the gurus mix these drugs, change them, or alter them with masking agents, the results are clouded and inconclusive, and fool the tester. Even some of the testers who are not fooled have to worry about lawsuits and proving a positive case if the matter goes to court. Unless the case is iron clad, it's usually not challenged in court. Some organizations have dropped drug testing altogether and surrendered the cause because of the lawsuit problem.

Almost all testing is done with urine, not blood. Most experts agree that blood testing is more accurate than testing urine, and that some of the drugs which are undetectable in urine can be found in blood. But blood has many problems, as it clots and spoils, has to be kept cold, and drawing it would be against the religious beliefs of many.

Also, most people just don't want to handle it because of contagious diseases, broken vials, etc. Blood is just a major

160

headache to deal with. It's also a lot more expensive, not to mention the possible civil liberties lawsuits, as taking blood is considered invasive to someone's body.

Many governing bodies may also fear that if they switch to blood testing the number of positive tests would rise sharply. This would hurt their public image, not to mention their big bucks corporate sponsorships.

The legal complications and fear of expensive lawsuits by the athletes have caused many drug tests to be a mere going-through-the-motions procedure. Many sport officials fear that some of the new drug testing methods may not stand up in a court of law. Drug testing is also expensive, so lower level competition can't afford it. Athletes could use drugs for several years before having to take a single test (at a high level competition).

Many bodybuilders can go for several years as they move up the ranks without ever having to take a single test. By the time that they have to be tested, they will have had several years of experience using steroids and will probably have learned the tricks of beating the tests. They may also be able to afford the more expensive stuff that can't be detected. The truth is, only the dumb ones get caught now. Unless you're one of the dumb ones, it's now fairly easy to take drugs and get away with it. Sadly, we can never again be sure that an athlete has prevailed by honest effort.

A few years ago, backstage at a major big-time bodybuilding contest, a bodybuilder collapsed and died suddenly. Because steroids were highly suspected as the case, it was largely covered up and did not get nearly the publicity that it should have. A few people on the "inside" believe that one day a bodybuilder will collapse and die on stage while posing. The drug problem will probably never get the attention it needs unless something dramatic like this happens.

There are many big-name bodybuilders who are now sick from steroid-related illnesses. Many have either died or will die sooner than they should have, because of drug abuse in the effort to get a trophy! In my opinion, true bodybuilding as it was originally intended, died sometime around 1960. And it has only got worse since then.

Bodybuilding and Physical Culture used to mean the same thing back in the pure and respectable days of John Grimek, Jack LaLanne and others in the forties and fifties. In the last forty years, almost every major contest bodybuilder and strength athlete has used drugs. Their pictures should not be on your gym walls. Take them down. These people should not be admired or followed. They are something to be ashamed of, and shunned. They are the arch enemies of Physical Culture.

MISCELLANEOUS THOUGHTS: PART I

May 2000

There are a number of topics which I get questions about all the time. I thought it would be useful to put them into article format, as they seem to be such popular subjects to many people.

Grip Work

Ask anyone who is serious about strength training and they will usually advocate the importance of grip work. It only takes a few minutes to fit it in—at the end of your workout, or during rest intervals. You do have time! If you're not currently doing grip work, find a way to fit it in.

The late Bob Hise II of Mav-Rik, who was a walking Iron Game encyclopedia (and who began his competitive Olympic lifting career in 1929), told me, "Everything starts with the hands. The first thing I do when I take on a new lifter is stress the importance of grip work. You'll never get close to doing your best without it. You need strong hands for every lift—even squatting."

I've several items at Whelan Strength Training made by Bob Hise, including a metal version of the Weaver stick which makes just a couple of pounds feel heavy!

Our Iron Game heritage is filled with stories that feature the old-timers doing serious grip work. Take, for example, John Davis' famous 365-pound axle lift, Bob People's deadlift of 725 pounds with an overhand grip, Al Berger doing pinch-grip chins from his 2 x 12-inch ceiling beams, Thomas Inch's one-handed deadlift with a 2.47-inch thick-handled dumbbell. Warren Lincoln Travis, with just his right middle finger, lifted over 600 pounds. John Grimek set the record in the Weaver stick lift with 11 pounds with his right hand. Ian Bachelor could crush metal beer caps between his thumb and each of his four fingers.

Vic Boff frequently talks about the importance of grip work. He was a champion at the art of finger twisting, which was very popular years ago.

Steve Stanko used to cut leather while making lifting belts for Bob Hoffman at York Barbell Co. One day, the knife slipped and he deeply cut the palm of his hand, putting the knife almost all the way through it. He had a big meet scheduled a few days later (in 1938), and everyone thought it would be impossible for him even to compete. It was a bad cut and took many stitches. He not only competed, but he won, setting a new national record. During the contest, according to Hise, the stitches broke and Stanko's hand was bleeding profusely. To "plug it up" he used a handful of chalk; and with his grip at half strength he still won! All that grip work paid off for Stanko. His toughness was typical of men of that era.

Try to avoid using supportive gear if possible—i.e., straps, wraps, etc. Make your hands hold the bar; they are the weakest link in your muscular chain. You should try to get them stronger. They will never get stronger if you use supportive gear. Supportive gear is not always bad, and sometimes helpful for certain people and specific situations. However, I believe that you should attempt to train without it if possible.

Thick-bar training will also aid your grip. If you don't yet have any thick bars in your gym, I strongly recommend that you add one, *but use it prudently.* Don't use a thick bar exclusively, but make its use *an addition* to your program.

I jumped on the bandwagon of the thick bar craze about 5-6 years ago, and even put thick handles on most of my machines. I've since removed them and now just occasionally put them on for a day of slow-rep training, but usually leave them off.

I learned through experience that it's more beneficial to do grip work separately, rather than mixing it in with regular work by using a thick bar for many exercises. When, for example, you perform rows with a thick bar, you "sacrifice" major body strength and growth for the sake of grip work. You simply can't lift as much weight with a thick handle on most lifts, so major muscle groups are "sacrificed" for grip work. But use a thick bar properly and it will be a great addition to your program.

The wrist roller is also a must and can be easily made. Use it two ways—palms-up and palms down. Consider implementing one or more of any specialist gripping devices into your program too.

You don't have to train to be another Rich Sorin or John Brookfield to reap tremendous benefits from doing grip work. Consistency is the key—an extra 10 minutes at the end of your workout, or even less if you use a thick bar, will reap tremendous benefits.

Multiple Sets or Just One?

This is one of the most argued about topics in strength training, and the answer is not the same for everyone. I believe you must train in a moderate to high-rep range to make one-set-to-failure for a given exercise work, as low reps require a lot more warm-up sets. With classic one-set-to-failure training, usually two (or just a few) warm-up sets are done to *start* the entire workout. One would be for the major upper-body exercise e.g., bench press, and one would be for the major lower-body exercises, e.g., deadlift. Then you move through the workout with all the training weights pre set and with little or no rest between sets/exercises. The rep range is high enough to have a built-in warm-up, but if you use lower reps you'll need more warm-up sets. Of course, individuals vary in their warm-up needs and Stuart, for one, believes that just a single warm-up set for (especially) the squat or deadlift is totally inadequate for many people, even if they use high reps in their work sets.

If you *truly train to muscular failure*, then one-set-to-failure works and is all you need. The problem is that many people, if not most, don't really train hard and don't understand what true muscular failure is. They think that they are going all out to failure, but they actually end the set far too early. *In my opinion, one-set-to-failure is not enough if you're not truly training hard.*

One set to failure is not fun. It's brutal and *uncomfortable.* I guarantee you that if you let Dr. Ken put you through a one-set-to-failure workout, you'll not be smiling at the end of it, and you'll not want to train for several days. Many people who claim to have tried one-set-to-failure have only given it a 90% effort, and then claim that it does not work. They have no clue. *One-set-to-failure definitely works, but you have to work your ass off to make it work.* You can actually get bigger and stronger than you've *ever* been in your life, with only two fifteen-minute workouts a week, *if* (and that's a big if) *you truly go all out.* Most people don't or can't.

It all boils down to this: The harder you're willing to work, the fewer sets you have to do, period. Sometimes it takes several months of training before someone learns how to give 100% and really go to failure. But some people never learn, partly because they really don't want to train to failure, and are not willing or able to endure what it takes to make it work. For these people, multiple work sets are better.

People are always asking Drew Israel how much time he spends training per week. But when he gives them the answer, they frequently refuse to believe him. Drew usually trains "Thirty minutes, tops" *per week* (exactly as I described in the opening paragraph in this section, including warm-up sets). He trains to true failure and is on the floor at the end of each workout. Most people are not willing to train like this and probably would do better with two work sets per exercise. If you're willing to do what it takes, however, one work set is a great thing.

Metabolic Conditioning and the Stamina Factor

Sometimes, for off-season athletes, I want them to do multiple sets to failure (two or three) because I don't just want to build muscle and strength, but also *stamina*. My goal is to train them even harder than they will be trained later on when they report to their camp. I want them prepared. I don't want them to run out of gas after 30 minutes or less. It usually takes around three weeks to get through my one-hour-multiple-sets-to-failure workout without feeling sick. *The human body can only take so much.* But it's not just the strength factor I'm concerned with, but overall body stamina factor as well.

To be able to stay on your feet for the whole one-hour workout is brutal. If you go down, you still try to get back up and finish the workout. If you do multiple sets to failure, you must be careful not to overtrain. This is where *the art part* comes in, and you use your instinct with regards to employing variety in the volume.

Weight Training, Calories and Cardio Work

You burn fewer calories with one-set-to-failure than multiple sets work, so you may have to put more emphasis on your cardiovascular training to keep your bodyfat down. Keep this in mind if you do one-set-to-failure and bodyweight keeps piling on. You'll build a lot of muscle and get stronger and stronger, but you'll be burning a lot fewer calories and may need to do extra cardio work to make up.

One-set-to-failure does work and will get you big and strong asyou can possibly get. It's a great thing, and can almost make you feel guilty because it take so little time. Drew and I joke about this all the time. But it's brutal and works only for those who do it right.

Remember, the harder you work, the fewer sets you have to do.

So-Called "Old Time" Training

Everything old is not always better as far as strength training is concerned. It was definitely better in the old days as far as the drug problem is concerned, but that's about it. For those of us who choose to carry on the physical culture traditions of our Iron Game pioneers, today is a far better time in many ways. Even though we're dwarfed by the mega-hype mags, there *is* a lot of good information available, probably more than ever! You just have to know where to look. It's our responsibility to spread the word about the good magazines like *Hardgainer*, the good books like the ones from CS Publishing, and the good web sites like Cyberpump!, Hardgainer, and NaturalStrength. There are also good newsletters, videos, etc., available. We also have far better (and more available) strength-training equipment, far more good gyms, far better nutritional knowledge, and far better strength and conditioning programs for athletes. We also have far better knowledge about general health—many of the old-timers smoked because they did not know any better.

There's also a popular misconception by some people about how the old-timers trained. There's a big difference between the old-timers and the old, old, old-timers. The old, old, old-timers (mostly pre-20th century and very early 20th century) may have mainly lifted things like rocks, anvils and bags of flour, because they had no options, but since Milo Bar Bell Company started mass producing the barbell in the early 20th century, 99% of training after this point has been done with barbells and dumbbells.

Look through all the old magazines and see how many pictures show barbells versus anvils, bags of flour and various other objects. (After Milo Bar Bell Company, odd objects were simply used to occasionally test strength and are actually far more popular today than they were then.) Almost all old magazine pictures will show barbells and dumbbells (in the photographs that are not posed). The old-timers improved on what the old, old, old-timers did, and we've improved on what the old-timers did. Look also at the thickness of the bars used in the old mags. For almost as far back as your collection will go, the handles were thin, not thick.

It's my opinion that odd-object lifting is misunderstood by some. Some people just like to collect odd objects. They are more concerned with the actual object than the movement they are doing. The object has become the center of attention. Who can find the most exotic, cool object? This has become a sort of competition for some people—the object itself has become the focus, not the movement or exercise. Keep your focus on the movement not the object! The object is not that important, and not worth collecting junk over. Progression is far easier to monitor with barbells, dumbbells and machines. It should not be the object that earns respect or shows how "tough" you are.

Twenty years ago, most machines were nothing but junk. Not anymore. Anyone who uses the blanket statement that all machines are junk now, or for wimps, is greatly misinformed, living in the past and just not up to speed. Today, we've some great machines available. Southern Xercise, Hammer Strength and MedEx make machines that give you many more options and the ability to work more planes of motion. These new plate-loaded machines are isolateral, balanced, smooth, safe, and are literally just guided barbells. Things change. Things improve.

Do you need to use these new machines to get optimum results? Of course not. A simple barbell will work wonders if you use it properly. It's all you really need to get great results, but *alternatives are available.* These options were not available to the old-timers. We're lucky to have these options!

I would bet that most of the old-timers would have loved the great machines that are available today. (The old-timers also used outhouses—does this mean that we should not use modern plumbing?) Keep the old-time stuff in perspective, and use the best information and equipment that you have available.

MISCELLANEOUS THOUGHTS: PART II

July 2000

Three-Days-Per-Week Whole-Body Training

Amazingly, many people who should know better are still fooled into thinking that more training frequency is better. They train by doing three whole-body workouts per week. This is a mistake, and too much if you're training hard. Cut down your whole-body workouts to no more than twice every week, and you'll feel a lot stronger and recovered for your training.

Most guidelines that recommend three-times-per-week whole-body routines are just for general fitness and "toning." They are not meant for serious strength training. These "toning" workouts are not heavy or high in intensity and are usually for the "Johnny Homeowner" sort of trainee who is just trying to "firm up" for the golf course.

If you train seriously, heavy, progressively and hard in a true high-intensity fashion, you would be far better off training with fewer than three whole-body sessions per week. The Whelan Strength Training guideline is twice every 7-10 days.

*Three day per week training can work well if you use much less volume or use the heavy, medium, light style as in the York courses where you are not going all out every time. If you use a higher volume, high intensity style with heavy poundages, multiple sets and cover your whole body including grip, neck, abs and calves for a one hour duration, two workouts per week are better than three.

Cardiovascular Exercise

There's been a lot of misinformation written recently about cardiovascular exercise. Unless you're a competitive strength athlete—usually in your twenties—you should be doing some sort of cardiovascular exercise. Even if you're competing in a strength sport, a minimum of 20-30 minutes three times per week should not hurt your strength much (if at all). The health benefits of keeping your bodyfat down and strengthening the most important muscle, your heart, should be enough reasons for you to be doing it. There has been some recent research which suggests that strength training is far more beneficial for your heart than previously considered. This is good news. But that does not mean that you should not stop doing cardio. Do both!

Many people are under the false impression that all cardio work is done slowly (at low to moderate levels of intensity), and for long durations up to an hour or more. This is not true. There's a wide range of intensity and duration you can adjust to suit your needs. You should design a cardio routine to fit your goals and personal enjoyment. Go on a Stairmaster and do a higher intensity interval workout for 30 minutes, and you'll see the light.

When it comes to information on cardiovascular exercise (and nutrition), I believe in taking a conservative approach. Most of the anti-cardio information (and nutritional quackery) is found in muscle magazines and is written by lay experts with no more than a hunch. The overwhelming opinion in academia, medical and sports research (from doctors and fitness experts who have actually been educated in the field), is that cardiovascular exercise is important and should be done by all who are able to do it.

I would much rather trust people like Dr. Ken Cooper than the anti-cardio crowd. For every lay expert that's anti cardio, you could easily find 100 professionals in medicine, research and academia who strongly think otherwise. Until these numbers are greatly changed, I strongly recommend you keep doing your cardio.

171

Zero- and Low-Carb Diets

To me, anyone on a zero-carb diet is just showing his stupidity. What fuel do you think your brain burns? Have you have heard of the Krebs cycle, energy systems, ATP or fast twitch (type IIb) muscle fibers? You can't have if you believe in zero carbs. When you strength train, you burn carbohydrates as fuel. Your body can't compensate for poor fuel. If you're out of gas and inadequately fueled, you're not capable of training hard and are doomed to fail. You can get all the rest and recovery you want, be mentally focused, and eat lots of protein, but you'll still feel weak and tired if you don't have enough glycogen storage in your muscles and liver. You'll not make it through your workouts. Complex carbohydrates are essential to your training success. Don't be fooled by the quackery.

If you don't believe me, go to a registered dietician for advice. Don't go to a health food store for advice. Don't read the mega-hype muscle mags for nutritional advice. Don't go to your gym for advice on nutrition either, as people there are no better. Don't ask a bodybuilder for nutritional advice. Don't ask your chiropractor for nutritional advice. Don't ask your bartender for nutritional advice. Don't ask a personal trainer for nutritional advice. See a registered dietician. Get it?

The Use of Supplements

If you're eating well, I don't believe you need food supplements for strength gains, but a good one-a-day type is a good insurance policy. Your emphasis should always be on food, but the one vitamin-mineral pill per day acts as your insurance policy and fills in the gaps of missing nutrients on a daily basis. A good vitamin-mineral pill is a wise move and not a waste of money. As far as protein powder is concerned, you definitely don't need it and can find far more efficient and cheaper ways to get enough protein. I recommend up to a gallon of skim or 1% milk per day and/or two cans of tuna per day for individuals in need of a protein supplement. This will give you plenty of protein, and probably too much when in addition to your three regular meals per day. *Supplements CAN be beneficial for your HEALTH (not cosmetic or strength gains). Things like krill/fish oil, time released Niacin, and vitamin D etc, but these have no real bearing on strength gains. Do your own research for supplements for health purposes.

Isolation Exercises

Some isolation exercises are not bad to do and can be a good addition to your program. I believe that the core foundation of your program should be the big basic compound exercises. That, however, doesn't mean that you should never do any of the isolation exercises. As long as you're not looking for the easy way out, and substituting the isolation exercises for the much harder multi-joint lifts, using a few of the isolation exercises in addition to your program can be beneficial.

Strategic Slow Training

I've recently been experimenting with various speeds of motion, and believe me folks, the slow stuff is tough. Anyone who says it's for wimps has not tried it. I've no problem with slow training itself, and respect it. I do have a problem with some of the dogmatic organizations and individuals who consider themselves the leaders of this type of training. They preach that you must train slow all the time, or you're scum. They claim that you're ignorant if you don't do it exactly like they say. In that case, everyone from Eugene Sandow, Alan Calvert, George Jowett, Peary Rader, Sig Klein and John Grimek, to Bob Hoffman and everyone in between, was ignorant to, right? Yeah, right!

Many training methods work, and this also goes for speeds of motion. I've recently used workouts with different speeds in the same session. I sometimes target problem lifts in a routine for slow training. Problem lifts are those that may cause irritation or have a history of bothering you in any way that's injury related. I've trained with a regular 2/5 speed on most exercises, but used a 5/5, 8/8 or even 10/10 speed on exercises that may bother an individual. For example, I've had many trainees who've had problems with the military press bothering their shoulders, and I change to a slower speed and they are fine with it. I've coined this use of slow training as "strategic slow training."

Deaths Are Not Good for Business!

I'm getting more and more visitors coming to WST who really have no business showing up. Most are from out of state and here on business or visiting the capital, and just figure they will casually stop by for workout while they are here. Many are in their forties or older, and clearly not up to the type of training normally done here.

They come with good intentions and are usually good natured, nice people; and I try to accommodate them and make them feel good about their visit. I usually require a two-hour orientation and a three-week conditioning phase for my regular local clients, so it's very difficult for me to have someone just walk in and train hard, especially if they are not in good condition. Of course I'm not going to train a 40-year-old stranger who I've just met as hard as I would a 22-year-old athlete I know. I pretty much just guide the visitors through the workout and try to make them feel good about it, and keep them on their feet. They may finish the impromptu workout, but they would never finish the standard planned workout.

Authors Update: I no longer train visitors without the orientation, and generally try not to train people without a minimum 3 month commitment.

MISCELLANEOUS THOUGHTS: PART III

September 2000

5-5-5 Training

For the last several months we've been doing a lot of this, and it's brutal. I got the idea from Tommy Metzger who performed a killer set on the Tru-Squat using this style at last year's Capital City Strength Clinic, as part of Drew Israel's segment. When he finished his set, Tommy could hardly walk. His knees buckled and he flopped around like a newborn calf trying to walk! no exaggeration. You can get a glimpse of this in the third Capital City Strength Clinic video. We use it on several machine exercises, but it's especially tough on the Tru-Squat.

To start the set, do a concentric motion for 5 seconds but don't quite lock out. You hold it in a static hold for 5 seconds. Using the Tru-Squat you have someone put the pin in the top hole after you've started down. You push against the pin in an isometric contraction at the top position for 5 seconds. Then lower the weight for 5 seconds, pause slightly at the bottom, and repeat. Get 5 reps like this and you'll be destroyed. WE add 5 pounds if 5 reps are reached in good form.

For upper-body exercises, which are not as demanding as the Tru-Squat, we add something further. In the Hammer Chest Press, for example, right at the point where you're getting stuck with the 5-5-5 and can do no more reps, you shift into regular speed to end the set. You can usually perform a few more reps at the end by doing this. I jokingly call this "double ecstasy failure." Though you try to come up as fast as you can, you can only move very slowly because your muscles are so fatigued. But you still lower the weight slowly. Just thinking that you can do the concentrics "fast" usually enables you to get a few more reps, even though you're not moving fast at all.

The 5-5-5 stuff is truly brutal and not for everyone. I pick and choose carefully when to use this and who to use it on. It's not something that we do all the time either, but for some individuals it's a productive (muscle shocking) change for a few months. Of course, ultra hard work such as this requires ultra prefect attention to nutrition and sleep, or else overtraining will result.

An Over-40 Success Story

Over two years ago Peter Elam came to the second CCSC and signed up for training at WST soon after. Peter was a 42-year-old beginner and never weighed over 149 pounds at a height of 5-7. He was also having problems with a shoulder he hurt in a car accident. He was getting physical therapy for it, and expected to get some insurance money because of the injury.

At first he was a little skeptical, but kept coming back and religiously got worked hard twice a week. He soon developed an appetite due to all the hard work, and it wasn't such a strain for him to eat all the food I told him to. Peter did everything he was told and the results began to show. If I told him to eat 5-9 pieces of fruit and vegetables per day, he counted them and did it. He never skipped breakfast, and ate three big main meals every day. He drank at least one half gallon of skim milk per day and, between meals, ate two cans of albacore solid white tuna packed in water.

I targeted his shoulders with strategic slow training for about eight months, using 8/8 speed. The rest of his workout was done at normal/regular speed. His shoulders responded so well that the insurance company will not give Peter the money he was supposed to get from the car accident. They now don't believe his shoulders were even hurt. I jokingly told Peter that I was sorry for costing him money; but he would rather have strong healthy shoulders, so he made out fine in the deal after all. Peter is now 44 and biologically about 10 years younger than when he started, and a whole lot stronger. He's now squatting close to 300 pounds for 10 reps, and deadlifting 375 on the Hammer Deadlift machine for 10 reps. He also weighs a solid 185 pounds. Not too shabby for a 44-year-old who started training at 42 with a bum shoulder.

Peter is barbell squatting because we use both free weights and machines. From 1990 to 1996 I used almost only free weights. From 1996 I gradually went to mostly machines. About 6 months ago I brought the barbells, racks and benches out from the moth balls. I missed some of the free-weights stuff, and the same routine with the machines all the time were getting boring.

For select clients we'll do both barbell squats and Tru-Squats, at different times. We also do other barbell exercises sometimes too. Most of the older clients do only Tru-Squats for their squatting, as I don't want a bar across their backs. We just have a little more variety now, that's all. Peter still does his Tru-Squats, and they are torturous! In fact, Peter developed most of his leg strength from the Tru-Squat.

An Over-60 Success Story

Art Brown was featured a while ago in the "You're Not Aging...You're Youthing!" article in *Hardgainer*. Art is now 64 and doing much better, and is actually training hard for 64-year old. Art is 20 pounds heavier and has doubled or even tripled his strength on most lifts.

When Art first started he was limited by arthritis and could only go down one hole from the top on the Tru-Squat with no weight on the machine, for about 10 reps. And that was a struggle. I made Art take long rests and told him, "Breathe deeply, Art, but above all...*breathe!*" He's now an inspiration to all at WST. As the months and years have gone by, we've slowly moved the pin down. Now art is going all the way to *the bottom*, with 55 pounds, for 13 reps.

It took many moths, but Art is now able to go all the way to the bottom on the Hammer Pullover too. He had a bad case of arthritis, and for months could only go about three quarters of the way down, but now has no problem with it. Art has built his strength up from 90 pounds to 170 pounds in the Hammer Pullover. His Hammer Chest Press weight was only 70 pounds when he started, and now he trains with 170.

Art walks around with a spring in his step, is much more mobile, much stronger, much more flexible, and has much more energy. He's biologically about 15 years younger than when he started. The benefits of strength training go far beyond just getting stronger. You're never too old to start. Good work Art!

Natural Blender Drinks

You don't need to waste your money on protein powder. Experiment with your blender and you can come up with many ways to get protein, as well as vitamins and minerals, in a convenient and cheap way. Here's a drink I like: Get your blender and throw in a handful of ice, a banana, some strawberries, raspberries, blueberries, and one small container of low-fat yogurt. Fill up the blender with skim milk. Blend it up, and drink. It's delicious, and easy to make.

Exercise Sequence

There are many old simplistic rules in strength training that are outdated and need to be revised. Most were thought of many years ago when few people actually lifted. A good example of one of these so-called rules is to lift every other day. The intentions of the rule were good, but it's just not accurate.

Another rule that falls into this same category, in my opinion, is that you should always work larger muscles first. If you're training hard, this rule doesn't make sense if you've a planned workout that you want to finish. At WST, if you followed this rule, your workouts would last about 15 minutes and the training would not be balanced, with many muscle groups left out. It could be squats, leg press (or deadlifts) and lights out, workout over. Even if you made it through this, you would be so impaired that your upper-body work would suffer and you would not be at your best. This is especially true if you do more than one work set. My philosophy on exercise sequence is that it's guided by priority. My priority is to get you through the workout and finish all the work, so the muscles get balanced training. Since my clients are charged on the basis of time, it's in their interests to get their training over as soon as possible but without compromising the quality of the workouts. Though most people don't have this pressure, most trainees would still benefit from getting their training done sooner.

I usually follow a push, pull and legs sequence with a minute or so rest given after the leg work, and no rest between the upper-body exercises. If you follow a push with a pull you don't need to rest. This allows for a built-in recovery for muscle groups, with an additional minute after legs. After the one minute rest we do neck, abs and/or grip. This is done by strategically placing easier exercises after the hardest movements, to provide additional recovery while not actually resting. It's just good time management, and provides the chance for quality effort for the whole planned workout. By the time you return to the chest press for your second set/sequence, you'll have had a long rest for that exercise while actually not resting much at all overall.

Here's an example of an exercise sequence at WST. Keep in mind that there's no typical workout at WST, because each program is individualized according to the individual client. WE usually, however, do two different workouts each week. This exercise sequence is for a client with recovery ability better than average. After 5 minute cv warmup to elevate body temperature, and a series of careful static stretches and warmup sets, he'd do (1) Hammer Chest Press, (2) Hammer Pullover, (3) One-Legged Hammer Deadlift, rest on minute, do side-to-neck on the Hammer Four-Way Neck machine, 1 set of 20 reps on the Jubinville crusher grip machine, and then repeat a second sequence of the main three exercises. After one minute of rest it's abs. During rests, drinking water is encouraged.

An alternative push-pull-legs sequence could be dips, iso rows, and leg presses, followed by rest, wrist roller, and then a repeat of the dips, rows and leg presses sequence. The above are just sequence examples and each example may be a full workout for some clients but only half the workout for others.

Ignore the Dogma

Like in most fields, strength training has its share of strange personalities. We've the "fitness Nazis," quacks, egomaniacs and would-be kings. It's too bad that many of the so-called leaders of certain strength training organizations or "movements" fall into one or more of these personality categories.

There are many ways to strength train that will work, and you should find what works for you. You should also find what you enjoy. There are certain truths that apply to all successful programs, but these are very basic. In a nutshell, train safe, progressively, eat well and get plenty of recovery, and then you should succeed. Strength training is a simple activity and the true leaders try to keep it train way. The phonies make it dogmatic and complicated.

The wide range of methods make this an activity that can always remain fresh and enjoyed by those who do it. The unhealthy attitude by many of the self-proclaimed experts and leaders in this field are causing great confusion among beginners, and having a negative effect on the field as a whole. Anyone who tells you that you must train in an extremely specific way with absolutely no flexibility, is a fool who should be ignored. Such rigid rules include speed of motion, rep ranges, using odd objects, only using machines or never using them, only doing one set to failure, only doing multiple sets, only doing split routines, only taking 20 or more days rest between workouts, or the necessity of doing power cleans, (or never doing them.)

Enjoy Your Training!

I've frequently written that you should *enjoy* your training. Enjoy the effort, dedication, camaraderie, sweat and work. Enjoy the journey and evolution of training progress. Be grateful to be healthy and bale to train hard. Life is short. There may be a day when you would give anything to be able to train hard again. Training enjoyment is one reason there are so many different training methods. People enjoy different things and are usually better at something they enjoy.

There are even some individuals who don't believe you can enjoy training *and* be successful at it. I've recently read on various web sites some pitifully negative information concerning this subject. I think some people just write to get their name seen, with no regard for the well-being of the people who read it.

I'm a positive thinker so it's easy for me to understand how you can work your ass off (and frequently feel very uncomfortable) and yet still enjoy it. Some people just have a generally negative and cynical view of training, and life as a whole. They are just negative people. I feel sorry for them.

People have died trying to climb Mount Everest, but they must have enjoyed climbing or they would not have risked their lives to do it. Ask marathon runners if they like to run, and they will look at you like you're crazy. Of course they love it! They are in pain doing it, but still love it.

My advice to you is to work your ass off and still enjoy your training. Ignore the negative cynics who want you to be as negative and miserable as them.

BOB WHELAN'S Q & A

November 2000

Q. *Please provide a summary of how you evaluate a new client to ensure that the program you put him/her on is appropriate, considering a range of different ages and physical conditioning.*

A. I've learned from experience that one of the most useful mechanisms for evaluating and screening new clients, is the telephone. I don't necessarily want to train some of the potential clients who call Whelan Strength Training. I would say that most of the individuals who wouldn't be considered appropriate for WST-type workouts are screened on the phone without my ever having to see them.

I jokingly wrote about this several years ago, and described it as the phone test, and this still holds true. There are many good ways to exercise and not everyone really wants to do the type of training we do here. That's fine. I just want to be very honest and be sure not to waste their money or my time. Many people are looking for general fitness and can just call any personal trainer for this. I don't do general fitness, full-blown rehab or general wellness tinkering. Nor do I want to specialize in geriatric training, energy work, or herbal new-age exercise therapy. I specialize in strength training, mostly for the able bodied (or semi-able bodied) with optimum strength and muscular goals the mission—drug-free strength and muscular goals of course! I don't try to get people to come in just to get their money. By being brutally honest, most of the clients who show up at my door are appropriate ones and really want to do this.

By appropriate clients I meant that they agree on a training philosophy roughly outlined in the WST Commandments:

Whelan Strength Training Commandments

1. Thou shalt train for strength, whole-body fitness and health; and do cardiovascular exercise and flexibility training as well as strength training.

2. Thou shalt not smoke, take illegal drugs or abuse legal drugs.

3. Thou shalt not use steroids or assist anyone in obtaining them.

4. Thou shalt be mentally focused and give 100% effort at every training session.

5. Thou shalt strive for progressive resistance, using good form, without excessive rest between sets, and use the fullest (but safe) range of motion possible.

6. Thou shalt primarily focus on the basic compound strength training movements—multi-join, no isolation—and train the whole body with equal emphasis on pushing and pulling. The training foundation is overhead pushing/pulling, horizontal pushing/pulling, and leg, hip and back pushing/pulling.

7. Thou shalt not seek shortcuts, miracle formulas or gimmicks, but instead stick to basic and sound information concerning training and nutrition, such as *Hardgainer, Brawn, Beyond Brawn,* and *The Insider's Tell-All Handbook on Weight-Training Technique.*

8. Thou shalt perform hard progressive strength training, and not toning, shaping or bodysculpting.

9. Thou shalt not train bodyparts but train the whole body (hard) usually about twice every -7-10 days.

10. Thou shalt not rely on mega-hype muscle mags for training or nutritional advice.

Once I've determined that prospective clients agree with my basic training philosophy and they *want* to do it, (or they may not understand it all but are willing to learn), I spend two hours with them in an orientation. During the first part of the orientation I have them fill out an *extensive* health history questionnaire. This questionnaire is very thorough and will ask for just about any illness, injury or disease they have ever had. It takes usually about 20 minutes to fill out, and sometimes longer. We discuss at length any red flag items that they mentioned during verbal follow-up questions (from me) about any cardiac problems, high blood pressure, knee, back or shoulder problems, etc.

After the orientation I give them a physical assessment. I measure their height, weight, blood pressure, bodyfat percentage and muscular girths. I document this information in their training folder which also contains a record of their training. After the phone test, health history questionnaire, verbal post-questionnaire interview and physical assessment, I can size up a person's stability pretty accurately. I can speed up or slow down the conditioning phase as well as make adjustments to the core training program based on this important information.

After this part of the orientation is complete, I answer all the trainees' questions about training. I previously asked them (when I talked to them on the phone, for the phone test) to bring all their questions, written down, to the orientation. After answering all their questions, I've a list of several items which I cover with them that include: what total fitness is, the relationship between energy systems and rep ranges, mental focus, good form, the importance of progression, proper breathing, definition of intensity as applied to strength training, cardiovascular training, stretching, nutrition, muscle mag hype and bull, myths and misconceptions about strength training, and the dangers of steroids. Sometimes we don't finish in two hours. Other times I may shorten it if the person obviously is already on board, ready to go, and passed the phone test with flying colors.

As long as the client is with the program as far as philosophy is concerned, I'll work with them. It takes most people about three weeks before they are able to do the regular planned workout at normal intensity. Some of the younger well conditioned athletes can go to full speed quicker, while others who are a lot older and in the 40-60 (or older) range can take a lot longer. I also cut the older ones a lot of slack because of the age factor. Their planned workout, of course will not be the same as that for a young athlete. I'm very careful with the over-forty clients, and progressively and *slowly* work them a little harder the longer they train at WST. Many things like odd-object lifting, farmers walks, fifties days, etc., will not even be thought of with the over-forty clients. A select few of them who really want to, but only after they have proven themselves with months of training with me, will be allowed to do some of the extreme things.

I consider all *prior* as well as *current* injuries, and limitations with range of motion, etc., when designing their program. I may do a limited rehab program such as for Peter Elam (mentioned in the last issue). I've an overall core philosophy of horizontal, vertical and lower-body balanced pushing and pulling planes. I sometimes adjust and tweak it with strategic slow training for problem areas, or I may avoid certain areas of the body or movements, and just work the non-injured areas for some individuals.

Q. *What's your opinion of singles?*

A. This isn't a cut and dried answer. For most people I wouldn't recommend singles. Singles can be productive for a seasoned lifter with a background in doing low reps. I wouldn't recommend them for a beginner or for anyone who is strength training just for strength and health but has no desire to compete in a strength sport. The same goes for an over-forty individual with no background in doing very low reps. I don't generally consider singles dangerous, just dangerous for people who are not prepared to do them, which is probably most people.

If you're not prepared to do singles, which is probably most people, you've a greater chance of injury. It makes no sense to take the risk when you can get great results by keeping your reps in a safer range. For experienced and seasoned lifters like myself, singles are not dangerous and can be productive, because my body is prepared to do them. My muscles and tendons have thickness from years of lower-rep conditioning. I'm also experienced enough to properly judge the weight that I'll be attempting. You don't just slap on plates that are way out of your league, just to try it. Any weight I attempt, I actually believe I'll get, or have a good chance of getting.

I've a powerlifting background and have done singles for years, and have never got injured doing them. That's just me. I make sure to do several warmup sets and pay special attention to do a slow eccentric motion. I wouldn't jump into singles after a layoff or right after a prolonged period of higher reps. If you plan to do singles, you should first spend several weeks of decreasingly lower reps, i.e., fives, threes and doubles, before attempting a single. I also don't believe in doing singles too often. I still do a lot of lower reps in my own training, but only try a single now and then.

Q. *Is a tall person who has to move the weight a greater distance than a short person more likely to overtrain?*

A. No. People are generally proportionate in bone and muscle. In most cases more muscle mass goes along with more bone mass. This can't be left out of the equation or you'll get an inaccurate result and basically an excuse. If it were true that tall people had a strength disadvantage, then NFL linemen would be 5-8, the world record holders in all the various strength sports would all be short too, women would generally be stronger than men, and we would get weaker as we grow from childhood to maturity.

Most of the strongest athletes in the world are over 6 feet tall. You can't just measure bone length and come up with a disadvantage. The taller person only has a disadvantage if he has the same amount of muscle as a shorter person. You must take into account the muscle mass or the potential muscle mass that the individual has. In general a 6-6 frame has a much greater potential to carry close to 300 pounds of lean mass than the 5-8 person does. The latter has nowhere near the potential of the former. If course, there are going to be individual cases where a person is lightly muscles as well as being tall with long bones. This just boils down to poor genetics and not just a height issue. Not all tall people are lightly muscles, just as not all short people are lightly muscled. In general, a larger fame has the potential to have more muscle.

You must compare similar muscle mass genetics to the frame, to make a height comparison fair. You can't assume that all short people have great genetics and large muscles any more than you can assume that all tall people are lightly muscled and have poor genetics. Most people are also a mixture of body types and are not simply based in one of three clearly defined groups (ectomorph, mesomorph or endomorph).

Q. *If you could only do one exercise for each major area, which exercises would they be to cover the whole body:?*

A. This is going to be a general answer that can be easily altered if need be. In the WST Commandments I refer to planes of motion to cover the body, not just exercise. A main horizontal push would be the bench press. A major horizontal pull would be a rowing movement such as the Hammer Iso Row, seated cable row, etc. A major vertical push would be the military press, and a vertical pull would be the pulldown or chin. The major lower-body movements would be the squat and deadlift, but other options, e.g., the Tru-Squat and leg press are also productive. And don't forget abs/weighted crunches, neck four-way machine, head strap or manual resistance, and grip work.

Q. *What do you think of negative-only exercise, and its values?*

A. I get this one a lot. I've heard from many people who claimed to get good results doing negative-only training. To be perfectly honest, I don't see the sense in doing negative-only training. It's imbalanced training. I like negative training, but not negative only. I've never done only the negative. I want to work the concentric movements too. It's a matter of muscular balance. Most functional movements in life are concentric in nature, so I'd no waste productive training time ignoring the concentric movements.

Q. *How can the ideal rep/set scheme be affected by body type? For example, compare a tall light-boned person with a short heavy-boned person.*

A. The first thing that must be done here is to define what's meant by "ideal." Ideal for what? Is strength the goal, or just general fitness? What are you training for? The training *goal* has the most influence on the design of your program.

Let's first discuss rep range. The goal of your training will determine the rep range, as energy systems don't change based on your bone length. If you're training for a marathon, you'll train differently than if you're training to be a football player. If you're training for a strength/power sport, you'll generally need to do moderate to low reps. This is especially true if strength defines your sport. You must tailor your training to your goal.

If you have a specific goal, there are certain training principles that must be followed regardless of your genetics. For example, if your goal is to be a powerlifter, it doesn't really matter what your genetics are, you must lift the most weight you can for one rep. You must do low reps in your training because of the goal for your training.

There are other factors, however, that must be considered and altered. Training volume can be adjusted based on genetics, the need to gain muscle mass or lose bodyfat, injury history, age and other factors. A hidden and often overlooked factor is the intensity factor. Many people will be quick to point out their poor genetics, but slow to point out their lack of hard work. Before you give yourself an easier workout, take a look in the mirror and ask yourself, "Am I really working hard enough?" I believe that in most cases the answer lies here. You need to train harder.

If you're one of the few truly overworked individuals who truly train too hard, always do the hard exercises, don't make excuses, never miss workouts, eat right, get enough sleep, don't drink too much alcohol, do cardio training, have a positive attitude, never skip training legs, eat enough good food, get enough protein, are able to look in that mirror and know that you can't work harder...*and still you're not getting results*, then try taking an extra day or two off, and reducing your training volume.

Cardio training, and diet, also must be adjusted for your body type and needs. Do you need to lose fat? Then you must do more cardio and eat less. You need the opposite if you're light boned, thin and need to gain muscular weight.

For the majority of people who don't fall into the truly 100% dedicated and overworked category, the general information you've been reading for years applies with no special consideration for you. I recommend training twice every 7-10 days and a training volume of one or two work sets per bodypart.

Q. *What are the most reliable indicators that recovery is complete or incomplete, and that another workout should or should not be taken?*

A. I don't want to be giving out excuses here. I'll not say that if you're just tired, to take another day off (even if you haven't trained for 5 days). You may be tired because you're sluggish and *need to train* to feel better! You may not feel like training and are looking for an excuse. You can't always go by your feelings. You must have the *discipline* to train when you feel tired after working all day.

I can see no reason for the able bodied to purposely train any less than once per week, *and I'm stretching it here.* I don't recommend training once a week. I personally feel it's too little training, but there are some people who I respect who are getting good results from it. Who's to say that they would get better results if they trained more frequently? We should not now be in a competition to find out how little we can train. There's a limit to recovery but there's a point where *deconditioning* and atrophy start, and recovery ends.

In general, my recommendation is if you're *sore*, don't train. You need to heal. I wouldn't train if I was still sore, and I would also get a minimum of three days' rest between workouts. There's a range of recovery that's acceptable and will not lead to *deconditioning*. There are some who train once a week with good results. I would say that this is the extreme length of recovery acceptable, and too much recovery and deconditioning for the vast majority of people. Again, for the vast majority of my time, my recommendation is two workouts in a 7-10 day period.

BOB WHELAN'S Q & A

January 2001

Q. *What advice would you have for someone wanting to set up a one-on-one training facility such as yours? What are the bare minimums for equipment and location, how do I know if I've the right qualities to train people, how do I attract clients, etc.?*

A. The first thing I would recommend is to get yourself as qualified as possible. When I saw "qualified," I don't mean by reading magazines or hanging around the gym more. It doesn't matter if you're the most knowledgeable person in the world about training. Unless you can convince others of it, you'll starve. This is now no longer your hobby, but your job as well. There's a lot of competition out there, and lots of people think they can do this.

Focus on *education, not certification*. Certification is the easy road that most trainers take. The gym-chain trainers who spend half their time handing out towels, cleaning the bathrooms and wiping down the equipment, all have certifications. The only requirement for most of these certifications is a heartbeat and a check that doesn't bounce! The fitness director usually has a fitness-related degree.

The first thing I would do is enroll in an exercise science/physiology program. Get a degree in a fitness or medical-related field, (e.g., exercise science, physical education, kinesiology, chiropractic, physical therapy, etc.). A degree in the exercise or medical field is 1,000 times more valuable than a certification. It will put you ahead of 95% of your competition, and is much more impressive when clients call you. (Even when you just start, you can, for example, say you're a university student in exercise physiology.) At the last count, there were over 150 fitness certifications in the USA alone. Most are basically worthless and require no academic prerequisite. You can be a high school drop-

192

out and still get certification. (The only certification that requires a pre-requisite is the CSCS one from the NSCA.) I would get the NSCA/CSCS (Certified Strength and Conditioning Specialist) certification and then not waste any more time with certifications. The CSCS is probably the most widely respected strength training certification (but a distant second to a fitness/medical degree).

By focusing on education, you'll also get some fringe benefits. All kinds of doors may open for you from the people you meet. I was fortunate to get a part-time job working at NASA headquarters as an exercise physiologist. This wouldn't have happened if I'd not been a graduate student in exercise science. You can also volunteer as a strength coach or assistant at a nearby university. You must pay your dues, and will probably not even be able to volunteer unless you have a degree in the field, or are at least a student in the field.

Don't expect to be paid at first, if you try to get a job as a strength coach, but if you volunteer you can get something to build your resume on. Remember that most of the top college and pro strength coaches, unless they have unusually lucky connections, have a degree in the field. For example, Dan Riley and Ken Mannie have degrees, and Ken Leistner had to go to school and take tough classes in chiropractic to become Dr. Ken.

You must live in a populated area or you'll probably not be able to do the one-on-one coaching full-time. If you live in a rural area, you'll either have to do this part-time or be forced to compromise your training philosophy to accommodate enough people to pay the bills. I'm fortunate enough to live in a heavily populated area, so I'm able to stick to a strict philosophy. I've enough people to be able to do this. I could never be a general fitness practitioner just to get someone's money. This is what I call a "fitness prostitute." I would rather stick to my philosophy, and get a part-time job if I had to.

If you can get a facility in a city, pick a good safe location near the subway, if possible. Location is important. If people are afraid to go there, you could have problems.

I would advertise in the local papers and plan to keep the ads ongoing.

You must have the passion and energy to coach. If you truly have what it takes, you'll make it work. I started out in a studio apartment and slept with the benches and barbells next to my fold-away bed. I worked at a part-time job for the first two years, while going to grad school to finish my exercise science degree. You don't need fancy equipment to start. It took me over 10 years of work to get the equipment I now have. I spent the first few years with only York bars and plates, and a few pieces of Jubinville free-weight equipment.

You should also figure out why you want to do this work. It will not be easy. You must have the passion to make it work. You must have the passion to get clients to train with you. If you really don't love strength training, and enjoy teaching and helping others, then don't do it. You'll be taking a big risk if you quit your current job to give it a go. If you have the right intentions and the requisite passion, then go for it. It's very rewarding and worth the effort, but make no mistake about it, it will take everything you've got to make it work. I recommend starting part-time (and keep your current job at first) and slowly build up your client base before cutting the cord and going full time.

Q. *What do you think of partial rep training that some power aficionados promote?*

A. If you're not training to compete in a strength sport, I wouldn't recommend you do partial reps. But if you're competing in powerlifting, for example, partials can be very helpful to break a sticking point, by focusing on the area of weakness.

Partial rep training is beneficial for some as an addition to a regular (safe) *full-range-of-motion* program. This is mainly for advanced trainees and/or for those training to compete in a strength related sport. For example, if you have a sticking point on your bench press, after your regular bench press workout is complete, set the pins on your power rack in the area of your sticking point. You can do partial reps in the power rack and work on your weak link.

I only recommend this type of work *after* you've already done your full-range work and not as a substitute for it. I disagree with those who advise doing partial reps as a regular and primary way to train. For most people who don't plan to compete in a strength-related spot and have limited time to devote to your training, focus on the basic full-range exercises.

Q. *What do you think of just performing on exercise a day, six days a week, rather than the same six exercises performed at a single workout each week, or two workouts of three exercises each?*

A. Almost anything is better than nothing, so you could possibly make progress on any of the above programs, even though I'm always suspicious of those who say that they are "making progress" as justification for sticking with a poor and usually too-easy program. They want to stick to it because it's easy, and will fight and argue to do so. They are usually training in cycles and starting so low in each that it's impossible *not* to make progress.

Or, they are doing the bare minimum to make a difference in terms of volume, frequency and intensity, but only slightly better than not training at all. You could possibly make progress doing almost any program. Doing only one set of just a few exercises once a week would produce progress when compared to lounging on the couch! It's easy to make progress when compared to doing nothing. Is it the way I recommend to get optimum results? No.

In my opinion, all of these programs are too easy and not complete for optimum results. I would not perform one exercise a day for six days per week. It does little for your metabolic conditioning, burns very few calories, and is disruptive for complete recovery. There probably will be overlap in various muscles of the body being worked on consecutive days. Theoretically, you could "push" one day, "pull" the next day and legs on the third day, and repeat. This could work, as there would be little overlap. Would I recommend this? No, but it could work. In my opinion, you would not get in good condition doing this and it's just not enough to work your whole body for balanced development.

Six exercises once per week is not enough training for optimum results, in my opinion. It would produce too much recovery and deconditioning, although you still could make some progress. It's really not too hard to make a little progress. The closest of the given alternatives to the one I'd recommend is the three exercises performed twice per week. I would recommend more volume than three exercises though. For optimum results for the able bodied, I recommend a core program of five exercises done for one or two work sets each, usually to failure. That's two workouts every 7-10 days. A horizontal push and pull, and a vertical push and pull in each workout, and at least one major leg movement in each workout, e.g., the squat (or a variation like the Tru-Squat), some form of deadlift and/or the Hammer Leg Press. (Be sure, however, not to deadlift more than once per week.) If you can, you should add abs, and grip and neck work too. You can get each workout done in less than an hour—including the neck, abs and grip—which is not too much of a price to pay for optimum results. If you're just starting out you may have to go with a shorter workout, but if and when you're physically able, this is my recommendation for *optimum* results not just minimum results.

Q. *For about 7 months I've been having pain in my rear shoulders*

196

that was brought about by snatches, and clean and jerks I foolishly began about a year and a half ago. I was 40 years old at the time. Recently it causes pain when I bench press or do heavy shrugs. The pain hits in the area where the traps and lats come together. What's the best way to rehab something like this? I'm also doing the 20-rep squat and deadlift routine so that I don't lose strength while resting my upper back.

A. Before I answer your question, I'd like to say that I would not recommend snatches, or cleans and jerks for someone your age, unless you're training to become an Olympic lifter or have a background in these lifts. However, if you just want to clean the weight to do your presses, or if you like doing power cleans and are proficient at them, then that's different—go ahead and do them. But if you've never done them and have no desire to be an Olympic lifter, there are just too many other better and safer ways to train the same muscles. Doing deadlifts and rowing would work the same muscles better and safer for you in my opinion.

I recommend you continue to train your lower body but take a full month off from training your upper body, and get an MRI scan. When you come back, start with a single "pushing" exercise and a single "pulling" exercise in each workout. Don't train with a "regular" speed of motion. This is the perfect time to use strategic slow training. Start with a rep speed of 8-10 seconds for both the positive and negative motions, and reduce your training weight by 50%. When you can do 2 sets of 5 reps in good form, add 5 pounds. If you feel any discomfort at all, reduce the weight and work back up slowly and don't try to add weight until you've performed several pain free workouts with any given weight. I've had great success with this approach as a rehabilitation method.

After a few months, try to work up the volume of your training by slowly adding a few more exercises so you're doing a vertical and horizontal push and pull. I would stay with the slow speed for about four months before going back to a "regular" speed. If you like training slowly, you could stay with it. It's probably the safest way to train.

Q. *I've been strength training at home for the last two years. For the first year or so, my progress was excellent. For the last several months I've been doing cardio training for an hour five days per week. I'm constantly tired. I stepped up my cardio work as an aid to help control my weight. Can my aerobic work be negating my strength and muscle gains?*

A. It's my opinion that almost everyone should be doing regular cardiovascular training unless you're competing in a strength sport. The cardio training recommended by the American College of Sports Medicine is a minimum of 20 minutes at target heart rate (which doesn't include the 5-minute warmup and 5-minute cooldown), and a maximum of one hour, 3-5 times per week. You're now doing the maximum, so I'd cut it down to a more moderate level. Try doing three 30-minute workouts instead.

It's true that the more cardio training you do, the more it can harm your performance in strength training. You can't be a good marathon runner and a good powerlifter at the same time, but you can be moderately successful at both cardio and strength training. There's a difference between training for performance and training for fitness. If you're doing your cardio training for performance, then your strength training will suffer more; but if you're doing your cardio training only for fitness, your strength will be affected far less. If you're strength training for performance—e.g., competing as a powerlifter—the cardio work may hurt your performance. Most people are not training for performance, such as competing in a strength sport, although they are competing with themselves to get stronger.

Strength training will also greatly aid in fat loss. The harder you strength train, the more muscle you add, and as you get your bodyfat under control, you can decrease your cardio work volume and duration to a moderate level as your basal metabolic rate increases. Every pound of muscle tissue that you add will result in a passive burning of about 35-50 calories for day. Over a period of time the added lean muscle will be even more beneficial for weight control than cardio work. For example, 10 additional pounds of lean muscle will result in an extra caloric expenditure of between around 350-500 calories every 24 hours.

I fluctuate cardio recommendations depending on the age, health, bodyfat percentage and goals of the client. If someone is young (20s) and healthy, but very thin and trying to gain weight, I may temporarily have them do no cardio training for a few months to help put on some muscle. I recommend the same approach if someone is preparing for a powerlifting contest. For the vast majority of middle-aged individuals (who are probably not competing a strength sport) a three-times-per-week volume for 20-30 minutes duration each time is my bare minimum recommendation, even for those who are thin.

What's the point of training? If health is an important issue, and it should be, there should be no questions that you must do cardio training (at least to train your heart), and anyone who thinks otherwise is a fool. The more of a problem you have with bodyfat, the more cardio training you should do. If you're fat and genetically inclined to remain so, you need to slowly and safely up the cardio to four or five days per week for about 45 minutes in duration per session, to keep the bodyfat under control. *Who cares* if you lose 10 pounds on your bench press! Would you rather have a heart attack? Once you get your bodyfat under control, then you can reduce the cardio training to a more moderate level.

My cardio recommendations also depend on the volume of your strength training workouts. With the current trend of trying to find the minimum amount of training, you'll burn fewer calories. If your workouts only last 15 minutes, you may have to do more cardio work if your bodyfat percentage remains a problem.

199

BOB WHELAN'S Q & A

March 2001

Q. *Is MedX equipment better than Nautilus gear? If so, in what way?*

A. This answer depends on a lot of things. No one company makes all the best machines. Even among the companies that make good machines, there's usually a problem with at least one of their pieces. Investigate machines by their individual movements rather than by manufacturer. Generally, Hammer Strength, Southern Xercise, MedX and some Nautilus (Power Plus and older models) are the best, in my opinion.

Why do you want a machine? Are you training using a slow speed or a more regular speed? Which Nautilus or MedX models (and years) are you talking about? Some of the earlier Nautilus are a lot different (and better in my opinion) than some of their later models. Are you talking about models that are plate-loaded or with a weight stack? Some of the earlier (Arthur Jones' models) were similar in construction to latter-day Hammer Strength machines.

I'll give my opinion on machines, but I'm not one to strongly advise you to get a certain machine—I'm mainly a free-weights guy. I started using machines due more to my business needs than for my own training needs. Machines are generally safer and more convenient than free weights when dealing with the public. Many people may never really need them for their own training. For over 25 years I got along just fine without any machines.

Don't confuse "latest" and "newest" with best. There are many individuals who seem to collect machines like some people collect stamps or coins. They are machine snobs and will constantly evaluate and size people up by what machines (or how many machines) they have. They are usually ignorant about the history of Iron Game, and consider barbells primitive. They get upset if their machines get scratched or banged too hard during use. Many of them would rather polish their machines than use them. I know a lot of these types.

I don't love machines, but I do love training. To me, a machine is nothing more than a guided barbell—no better, no worse, depending on the individual using it. Once I find a machine that suits my needs, I usually keep it. I don't care about "newest" or "latest," or if it gets a few scratches. Many new models are not improved at all, but are actually regressions from former models.

You usually lose money when you sell a machine and purchase a replacement. You need time to get comfortable with a machine. Many people change machines so often that their motor learning and comfort level of using the machine is never fully optimized. For me, as long as my main training planes of motion are met in safe and natural movements, I'm happy with given machines and I'll probably keep them. Under these conditions there's no logical reason to trade a machine in. You also get plenty of variety with mixing free-weights into the planned workout, changing speeds and rep ranges, etc.

One of Nautilus' best recent lines was the plate-loaded Power Plus line, which I believe was discontinued a few years back. They made the best military press unit and I was lucky to get one before that line was discontinued.

You can't make a general blanket statement that one company is better for all machines. I love Hammer Strength machines in general, and own several of them, but I didn't like their behind-the-neck press unit I bought a few years back. I sold it because it had a floppy seat. My clients would slide down it when pushing, and thus have poor support. I called Dr. Ken and he told me, "Get the Nautilus Power Plus Military Press unit before they stop making them." I did and got one of the last models made. It works great, is heavy duty and compact, with a great natural and smooth movement. I would not have even considered Nautilus if not for Dr. Ken's advice. This is the only Nautilus piece I currently own, but I love this unit.

Choice of machine brand can be influenced a lot by your training quarters, including the space available. I love the machines made by Southern Xercise, e.g., the Tru-Squat, but their stuff is so big that I can only afford to take up space with a few of their pieces. If space was no option, I'd get more, but I'm paying a premium price (per square foot) for business rent in the heart of downtown Washington, DC, and have to conserve space to afford to do this. I have to get bang for my space.

I've a number of considerations when considering a purchase, e.g., quality of movement, space requirement, price, and amount of use. I have a variety of machinery including some combination units. Different people can have different reasons for getting certain machines.

One of the most important but rarely thought of questions is, "Can I move it into the allotted space?" This is something I've learned the hard way.

When I bought the Tru-Squat, several years back, I remember talking to Larry Nichols at Southern Xercise about delivery. Larry told me, "Don't worry about a thing; we'll have the United Van Lines truck come drop it off and it will be a snap. A 10-year-old could put it together! Will it fit in a tight staircase? No problem. Piece of cake!" Some piece of cake! Here's the rest of the story.

The United Van Lines truck came in the pouring rain and the driver was alone. The Tru-Squat was in a heavy-duty wooden crate, weighed a ton, and was more securely packaged than military equipment going to the Pentagon. The driver wanted no part of helping me break it down and carry the pieces in. I offered to pay him but he had other things to do. He used the hydraulic lift to lower the crate onto the sidewalk. Here I was in the rain, with a crate that weighed a ton, in the middle of a busy sidewalk in downtown Washington, DC. I managed to take the crate apart with a sledge hammer and chisel without injuring anyone. I then moved each piece of the Tru-Squat into the hallway lobby of the building at 800 7th Street. This took over an hour. Now, how was I to get it in the gym?

After realizing that the Tru-Squat came in only a few pieces and couldn't be condensed any further, I knew I'd have problems. I had doubts I could get it into my place due to the narrow twisting staircase that goes to Whelan Strength Training. I called a few of my strong clients to come help me. We scraped and gouged the walls for about four hours. It was getting late, and we were still a long way from being able to move the machine in. We'd already messed up the walls big time, but it wasn't enough. I got out a big saw and blindly cut out a huge piece of wall that adjoined the staircase and was blocking entry. I prayed that I would cut no wires or vital support beams. I was lucky. Then we soon got it in. Ecstasy! But we'd done serious damage to the aesthetics of the building. I called my landlord and said, "Glenn, I've got something to tell you. I was afraid you might say 'no,' so I went ahead and did it without asking..." Luckily, he worked out a generous deal to fix the walls! Here's the moral of the story: Make sure you can get a piece of machinery into your place *before* you go buying the gear.

Speaking of space, at WST, I've expanded and now have about a third more room. I'm below a Starbucks Coffee Shop and they had a storage room next to WST for years. Last year there was a fire here which almost put me out of business. Thank God for sprinkler systems! Starbucks recently expanded upstairs, and the storage room became available to me. As of October 2000 I picked up this place and now have three rooms at WST.

I brought out several old Jubinville pieces from storage and we now have more equipment balance.

To sum it up, according to Drew Israel (who is a machine aficionado), in general, I repeat *in general*, if you're training using slow reps (and have a lot of cash to burn), MedX is no question the best overall brand to buy. MedX gear is designed for slow training and the movement on them is smoother than on other gear. They are also very, very expensive; and you may need a demolition crew to get them in.

For my use, I don't consider the alleged slight improvement in a smoother motion (using slow speed) a good enough reason to change my equipment and lose a lot of cash in the exchange. This is especially so when you consider that I usually don't train using very slow reps. If you never train using a very slow speed, the smoother qualities of the MedX gear don't really make sense (or matter). Any of the big three machine manufacturers—Hammer Strength, Southern Xercise and MedX—along with some Nautilus, could serve you well as long as you're comfortable with the movement of the machines.

Q. *Do you feel that specific neck and grip exercises need to be included in a training routine?*

A. First, let me ask, "How serious about training are you?" Ideally, everyone should work grip and neck, but many people don't have the same passion for training, goals, needs and knowledge that I have, and only want to dedicate a minimum of time to training.

If you're an athlete (especially one involved in contact sports such as football and hockey) there's no excuse not to work your neck. In fact, I wouldn't train one of these athletes if he refused to do neck work. It should be a top priority for them.

A middle-aged businessman should also work his neck, and do some grip work, but if he is only willing to spend a given amount of time for training, he needs to try to get as much of his body worked as possible in the time permitting. Many women will not do neck and grip work no matter what you tell them, but they do train hard otherwise.

In the real world, sometimes neck and grip work gets sacrificed by some trainees, which is not the ideal training outcome but as long as they are getting the major muscles worked, trainees will still benefit greatly, albeit from an imperfect program.

Q. *I'm approaching 50 years old, and have been training for 30 years. What are some training goals to aim for?*

A. I can't give you specific goals without knowing more about you, but your situation sounds a lot like mine. I'm 46 and have been training for about 35 years. Since you have 30 years of training behind you, your situation is a lot different than if you were a 50-year-old beginner. First of all, never, *never*, ever surrender to age. You have a chronological or numerical age you can't change, but your most important age is your biological age. You can change and slow down that.

If you've been training for 30 years you're probably still biologically in your early to mid thirties, which is where I consider myself to be. You can get younger or older (to a certain extent) depending on how you take care of yourself. Look at Jack LaLanne and Vic Boff. Do they surrender to age?

I get people who come into WST all the time who say, "When I was your age, I could do this stuff, but I'm 40 years old."

I reply with, "I'm older than you. Quit talking about your age unless you want to be old." You should still try to increase your strength and muscular size for many more years before you settle into a comfortable maintaining mode. You have 30 years of training behind you which will benefit you greatly for the rest of your life. Things are far easier for you than if you were a beginner at age 50.

The main age-related things I give extra focus on are cardiovascular condition, following a healthy dietary plan, and avoiding injuries. Generally, you may need more warmup sets and less work sets than when you were in your twenties, but you can still aim to increase your poundages. Pay extra attention to using good form while training. I definitely need a day or two more recovery time between workouts now than I used to, and I put a lot more emphasis on sleep.

I can no longer eat whatever I want, without getting fat. When I was young I was skinny and had to eat two cans of tuna a day and drink a gallon of whole milk as well as eat a lot at normal mealtimes. I always seemed to be eating. I got used to this sort of eating after a while, and considered it normal. The problem is that when you get to your late thirties and early forties (earlier for some people), your metabolism definitely changes. You must eat less when you get older. If I continued to eat like I did in my twenties, I'd weigh 400 pounds now and would need to call Richard Simmons and the fire department to get me out of bed.

Q. *Bob, how is your training going? What are your goals?*

A. I strength train twice in a 7-10 day period. For the last few years I've been doing usually one or two work sets to failure per exercise. I usually do neck, abs and grip at every training session (time permitting), and do the following core program:

Workout A

1. Incline Press
2. Hammer Iso Row
3. Shruggs
4. Military Press
5. Hammer Pulldown

6. Barbell Front Squat

Workout B
1. Nautilus Behind Neck Press
2. Hammer Pullover
3. Curl with 2-inch-thick barbell
4. Dips
5. Chins
6. Deadlifts

Some goals? To keep getting stronger, stay young and injury free, lower my bodyfat a little more, never surrender to age, and just keep at it as long as I'm alive, like Vic Boff. More specifically, I want to front squat over 300 pounds for 20 reps (I'm getting close), and (tongue in cheek) get so big that people cross the street when they see me coming. Seriously, since I'm not powerlifting anymore, I just want to enjoy training get stronger, feel young, healthy and energetic, and add weight to the machines and bars I use.

Q. *What do you think about the effectiveness and safety of static contraction training techniques?*

A. Drew Israel has been experimenting with static contraction training. He claimed to get great results by holding a repetition at the midpoint of the range of motion, for about 40 seconds. This is all he did for a few months on all his exercises, for one "set" each, with no additional work. Drew would hold the machine in a mid-rep static position, and if he could hold for 45 seconds he would add weight next time. It was purely measured by time under load, and no reps were done. This is not isometric as some people describe it, because it's progressive and not against an immovable object.

But Drew is not the everyday type of guy. He's 6'4'' and close to 300 pounds of muscle, and extremely strong. He's been training for decades. I would not use the static-hold stuff for a raw beginner, for elderly or extremely out-of-shape individuals, or for rehab people.

If you're able bodied and healthy, and past the beginner stage, you could give it a try if you're so inclined. We've done some static-contraction training at Whelan Strength Training, with 5-5-5 training where each rep takes about 15 seconds, with 5 on the concentric, 5 on the eccentric and 5 on the static hold. It's very tough and good for a change of pace; but I wouldn't do it for more than four months or so. Once in a while, for certain clients, we'll do it the Drew Israel way, as a change of pace.

BOB WHELAN'S Q & A

May 2001

Q. *What would be a suitable way of attacking a sticking point or plateau in training progression?*

A. My opinion is that a sticking point is usually more mental than physical. There are many ways to battle a sticking point. I'll list some ways that have helped me.

When I was competing in powerlifting I would never let myself get crushed with the same weight more than two or three times in a row without making a change. If you keep failing with the same weight, it has a negative effect on your confidence and expectations. You can start o subconsciously expect to fail, and your confidence is destroyed. I frequently used this tactic on the bench press, which was my most mind-affected lift. I would constantly change the rep range and goals of sets. I would do each set instinctively. Let's say I got 4 reps with 315 on the bench and I couldn't get the goal of 5 reps. I would skip 315 altogether for a few months. Instead, for example, I would do as many as I could with 305, and then try for 3 with 335. Next workout I may have gone for 295 for 8, and 345 for 2. I would keep changing the goals for the set, and keep my mind positive and fresh.

Back in 1975 I was stuck for a long time at 295 on the bench press, and it seemed I would never get 300 (for a single). I was 21 and in the Air Force at the time, and training at the Castle Air Force Base gym, in California. My confidence for 300 was destroyed as I'd failed continuously for months. The big round number of 300 was really playing with my head, partly because I wanted it so badly. Finally I said, "The hell with it, let's go for 305! What have I got to lose!" I put 305 on the bar and felt no negative pressure because I'd never tried this weight before, and the previous failures with

300 were erased from my mind. It flew up like a rocket! Sometimes, adding weight to a goal is what's needed. You have nothing to lose, and a built-in excuse if you don't get it—because it's above your expectations already.

The key for me was to learn to stay positive and find ways not to let previous failures get into my mind. A good hitter in baseball, after striking out, will dwell on getting a hit the next time he faces the pitcher, and not dwell on the strike-out that just took place. I also developed defensive measures that I call positive rationalization. If I had a bad performance, I'd find a way to make it positive in my head.

If you're doing higher reps to failure in your training, change the poundage and goal for the set, which will change the rep range. You could also change the rep speed for a while, which will get your mind on a whole new goal, erase previous failures, and get your focused on working and not on numbers. This is one reason why I use what I've coined "Common Sense Periodization" every four months or so—a change in goals are needed to stay fresh. See my article on this in issue #61.

You could also put some positive pressure on yourself by getting a training partner who will push you, or by hiring a coach and training in an environment like at Whelan Strength Training.

Finally, examine your mental fundamentals. You must do more than just stay positive. Being only positive (but passive) will not work. Besides staying positive during training, you must learn to channel anger into your mental focus while lifting. Not enough information is written about this, which is a shame. You should have the mind of a "disgruntled postal worker" or psycho killer when you attack the bar. You should be temporarily insane, in a "going to war" state filled with anger, hate and rage aimed at the bar as you lift the weight. You must learn to manufacture this if you can't find it in yourself, just as athletes do (football players in particular).

You should never lift right after talking. Much is written about not talking during workouts. Many writers just say "Don't talk," but this isn't realistic. In real life, almost all trainees, unless they train alone, do talk to some extent during workouts. The key thing is that at least 20 seconds or so before lifting the bar, sop talking, clear your head, and focus on what you're about to do. Never go right from talking to lifting, or you'll be sure to fail.

Q. *I've read that you competed in powerlifting.* When did you compete, and what were your best lifts?

A. I competed for seven years from the mid seventies to early eighties. I usually lifted in the 181-pound class, but occasionally was unable to get under 181 pounds and would lift in the 198-pound class. I competed mainly in US military meets, and some open meets in Germany where local nationals were able to compete too.

I was stationed in Germany at Spangdahlem Air Base, not far from Luxembourg. Bitburg Air Base was only about 10 miles away (located in the town of Bitburg, where I lived in an apartment off base). I used both base gyms but trained mostly at the Bitburg gym since it was closer to where I lived. During that time there was a lot of lifting talent stationed in the area. Such notable lifters as Willie Bell, Russ Lewis, Harry Cook and Glenn Pieschke were stationed there at that time. WE learned a lot from each other and had a great training environment.

I had some of the hardest workouts of my life with Glenn, in the late seventies, in the dumpy Bitburg Air Base gym. I frequently had breakfast with Willie Bell, who got a waiver from the base commander to have as many eggs as he wanted at the chow hall. He frequently got a whole dozen eggs at once for breakfast.

Sports were taken seriously there, to keep morale up while away from home. Each base had a tackle football team and played other bases in front of large crowds. It was similar to small college level, in talent. There were several varsity sports in addition to tackle football, including powerlifting. I actually flew in a C-130 and officially got off work to go to Aviano Air Base, Italy (not far from Venice), for five days just to lift in a military powerlifting meet. It was great!

The first few years I had to struggle just to place, but I kept training hard and 1979 I would win all the time. At a bodyweight under 181, I deadlifted 555 in a meet in 1980. My squat was slightly over 500 and I had a double-bodyweight bench press of 365 (in training) but a best of 350 in an actual meet. You can frequently lift more in training because in a meet, strategy is involved and you don't take chances if you know what you need to lift to win. I've never owned or used a lifting suit or bench shirt. I did all my competitions in a simple wrestling singlet. My best total in the 181 class was slightly under 1,400. If I had a supersuit and a bench shirt like they have now, I could have easily totaled over 1,550 in the 181 class. Add drugs and I could have done 1800.

I actually totaled over 1,400 by best lifts. If you took my best lift in each of the three movements, and put them together, it would have been well over 1,440, but I never did my best lifts in all three in the same meet. You are also safer in a meet and just lift what you need to win.

I was crazy back then and would really get psyched-up at meets. I remember when the movie "Rocky" first came out, and raw eggs were cool because Rocky drank them from a blender. I wanted to "one-up" Rocky, so I ate raw eggs shell and all, and just chewed them right from the carton! To put on a show, I'd gargle with an egg, let some run down my face, and then chew it up. It looked like I was chewing gum. I used to go through several eggs during powerlifting competition. It would psyche the competition out. I wouldn't, however, recommend this to anyone, as raw eggs can make you very sick. I won't be doing this again! I was young and crazy back then, and lucky it never bothered me.

In 1983 I was also the base's powerlifting coach. In order to fill all the weight classes, which is the key to winning, I stood in front of the base post office for days, and watched everyone come check their mail. I was on a "midget hunt." I was looking for smaller people to fill the lower weight classes. I figured everyone on the base would check their mail, so I was patient and kept checking everyone's size as they came in. I would walk up to total strangers and ask them to come meet me at the gym later. I would teach them what to do, and some individuals who had never lifted in their lives got trophies because they had no competition! Boy, what a trophy will do for some people! Their self esteem totally changes. Once these 114, 123 and 132 pounders got their first trophies, they were gung-ho and became lifting fanatics!

The Spangdahlem Powerlifting Team had a bit of a dynasty going at the time. We won the CSC Championship for three straight years—1981, 1982 and 1983. Continental Sports Conference was for all the bases in central Europe, mainly from Germany. An all-star team was picked for the USAFE (US Air Force Europe) Championship from the best lifters from the CSC bases. The CSC all-stars competed against the UK Conference all-stars and the Mediterranean Conference all-stars (Turkey and Spain) for the USAFE title. I coached the CSC all-stars to the USAFE title in 1983.

I stopped competing because more and more I saw drugs creeping their way into the scene. Even in military meets, people were having drugs shipped to them in the mail, as well as buying them from the German economy. It made me sick. I saw a guy go from a 335 bench to a 410 bench in a matter of three months! He also fell back down like a rock as soon as he got off of the drugs.

Q. *What's the youngest age you'd recommend someone take up* training?

A. I started training at age 10, but I didn't get my first barbell set 'til I was 13. For three years I did a lot of pushups, chins/pullups, situps, leg raises and some dynamic tension stuff I learned from borrowing the Charles Atlas course from a friend. I mostly did the dips between chairs from the course, and got up to 200 a day. I made a wrist roller from a broom handle and some twine, and tied a brick to it. I also lifted pipe and scrap metal that my father had brought home from work to store in the basement before he sold it to a junkyard. My early workouts were usually done for high reps.

I think age 10 (for me) was okay because I loved it and wanted to do it, but for most people it would probably be too young. Unless the kid loves training on his own, don't encourage him to train 'til he's a little older, at least in his early teens. Even then, don't push him too hard, and don't make it overly serious. Encourage calisthenics when kids are very young, before they move up to barbells. Keep it light and fun at this early age. Training for pre-pubescents and pubescents must be supervised, as their bones are still growing. The rep ranges should be kept high for these youngsters—*NO LOW REPS OR SINGLES* for them while they are still growing.

Q. *How do I bring up a lagging bodypart?*

A. I would continue with my regular well-balanced routine with equal emphasis on pushing and pulling from the horizontal and vertical upper-body planes, as well as that pushing and pulling for the lower body. I would be sure to get all my neck, abs and grip work done too. When the balanced, planned workout has been completed, then I would spend some time on a few extra sets for the lagging area.

Q. *How would you rate the front squat, and what would be* considered a "heavy" poundage, say relative to *400-pound* conventional squatting?

A. I've always like front squats and have done them for years. I even did them exclusively for several months when I was powerlifting (as an experiment), and was able to convert to the full squat easily, without losing any strength at the next meet. I don't know any formula for comparable numbers, and could be way off for some people; but I would consider a front squat of 300 pounds for 20 reps similar in difficulty to 400 for 20 in the regular (back) squat.

I've recently started front squatting again after not doing them for several years. They fit like a glove! I use the crossed-hands method and never put a board under my heels. About ten years ago I hurt my knee using a board. It was about the size of a 2 x 4, and I felt a sharp pain in my knee. I had trouble even walking for several weeks. Luckily, nothing was torn, just strained. I had to cease all leg work for about six months, that's how bad it was hurt. Don't use a board, or you're asking for trouble. Be sure to use a power rack, as you don't want the bar landing on your thighs if you lose control of it.

You must be patient with this exercise, as it takes a while to get our balance and feel conformable. I think it's a better indication of leg strength than that back squat, because you can't use techniques like having the bar very low on your back, or leaning too far forward while coming up. You must say upright when front squatting or else you'll be forced to dump the bar.

Q. *I've heard that lifting weights crea*tes endorphin release within the body. But after training I sometimes feel mentally depressed, *even though I've had a good lifting session. What's up?*

A. I'm not a mental health expert and probably not qualified to answer this except to tell you that your problem sounds like depression. I would work on building a positive attitude foundation. Buy *The Magic of Thinking Big* by David Schwartz, and work on your attitude. Get involved in the spiritual side of your life too. If you continue to feel depressed even though you're doing everything you can for yourself, seek out a clinical psychologist who can help.

Q. *Which is the better, squat or deadlift?*

A. Ideally, neither. You should do both unless you have medical reason that prohibits you from doing them. There are pros and cons of both lifts, and it makes no sense to argue which is so-called better. To be balanced in strength, I would always recommend a variation of both, done once per week each. If for a medical reason you can't do one of them, you can be very well saved by working on a variation of either lift.

Q. *If knee and back injuries prevent heavy squatting and deadlifting, what can I do instead in order to gain?*

A. If you have a good leg press like a Hammer Strength or MedX model, you have a very good alternative. I say a "good leg press" because the type of leg press model makes a huge difference. Many commercial gym leg presses are junk. They are way too easy and the average grandmother can use about 500 pounds on them and still not break a sweat! They are on a sliding sled and you have to use all the weights in the gym to get enough resistance to have a hard workout.

Q. *How important is thumb strength? I use a grip machine but it only seems to work my fingers other than my thumbs. Should I be doing some pinch grip work as well?*

A. Your thumb is extremely important for grip strength, and acts as a stabilizer. It's still working hard in a static contraction even though it's not moving like the other digits are. You should work the grip in both the crushing and pinching motions.

The grip machine is a unit for building crushing strength. Pinch grip work should be added to the program. This could simply be done by pinch-gripping barbell plates, or you could buy a purpose-built device such as the "Titan's Telegraph Key" from IronMind®, which we use all the time at WST.

BOB WHELAN'S Q & A

July 2001

Q. *I like to do sprint triathlons from June to August (one per month), but don't want to waste away. How can I continue to weight train without overtraining?*

A. Any type of athlete, whether a triathloner, football player or whatever, should continue to strength train during the actual competitive season. Many athletes make the mistake of being at their strongest before the season starts, gradually get weaker during the season, and are at their weakest at the championship game! By not training during the actual competitive season, they are also more prone to injury as the season progresses. You should not be at your strongest and most physical ready state before the season. IT should be the opposite. You should continue to get stronger as the season develops. You should not be satisfied to just maintain, but continue to train focusing on progression during the season. Even if you usually don't train using one set to failure, during the season is when it's extremely beneficial.

If you have one of those Neanderthal coaches who tells you to stop strength training during the season, you should secretly do the strength training on your own. You must take care of yourself and not let the foolishness of others hurt you. Everyone else will be getting weaker and will be shocked at how fresh and strong you are at season's end.

What's the point of training for your sport if you're not going to reap the benefits from it? Of course, you must greatly reduce your training volume during the season, but you should still continue to train with hard and progressive albeit much shorter workouts. You may also have to train less frequently. You're going to be zapped by all the regular sport work and need all the rest you can get in order to have a good performance. You want the strength training to aid your performance, not hinder it.

218

I recommend that you train you whole body once every 4-5 days with weights, or two workouts in a ten-day period. Each workout should only take about 20 minutes to complete, using just one set to failure in the core movements using moderate to high reps. During the season, do *only* the core exercises; save the isolation movements for the off-season.

Here's a good example of a one-set-to-failure routine during the triathlon season:

1. Bench press
2. Horizontal row
3. Pulldown or chin
4. Military press
5. Major leg movement

By a major leg movement, I mean the barbell squat, Tru-Squat, leg press or deadlift. I recommend you alternate the squat and deadlift—i.e., do each just once every ten days. If you're in a contact sport like football or hockey, I would continue to work the neck in-season also.

Q. *As one ages, what proportion of training time should be devoted to weight training, aerobics and stretching?*

A. The strength-training requirement is similar to that given in the previous question, about athletes' in-season training. As you age, you should cut down on your volume and frequency a little, depending on how you feel. I strongly recommend one set to failure and slow training as you get older. Keep training progressively and hard, with short workouts and plenty of recovery, for as long as you're physically able!

I advocate devoting at least three days per week to cardio training, for both young and old trainees. The minimum standard requirement of the American College of Sports Medicine is three, not two days per week! As one advances in age, cardio work is definitely increasingly important and more of a life-and-death issue.

I fluctuate the cardio recommendations depending on the age, health, bodyfat percentage and goals of the client. If someone is young (20) and healthy, but very thin and trying to gain weight, I may have them do no cardio training for just a few months, to help put on some muscle. If someone is preparing for a powerlifting contest, then the same thing. For the vast majority of middle-aged individuals (who are probably not competing in a strength sport) a three-times-per-week frequency for 20-30 minutes' duration is the bare minimum, even for those who are thin. What's the point of training? If health is an important issue, there should be no question that you must do cardio training (at least to train your heart) and anyone who thinks otherwise is a fool.

The more of a problem you have with bodyfat, the more cardio training you should try to do. If you're fat and genetically inclined to remain so, you need to slowly and safely up the cardio to four or five days a week for about 45 minutes in duration each time, to keep the bodyfat under control. Who cares if you lose 10 pounds on your bench press? Would you rather have a heart attack? Once you get your bodyfat under control, then you can reduce the cardio training to a more moderate level.

The issue of cardio training is one of my pet peeves. There has been a lot of misinformation written recently about cardiovascular exercise. Unless you're a competitive strength athlete, (usually in your 20s), you should be doing some sort of cardiovascular exercise. Even if you're competing in a strength sport, a minimum of 20-30 minutes three times per week should not hurt your strength much if at all.

There has been some recent research which suggests that strength training is more beneficial for your heart than previously considered, but that does not mean you should now stop doing cardio. You should do both! Strength training is not enough by itself to meet the demands of cardiovascular fitness. Much of the erroneous anti-cardio information has been put out by the slow training cult.

Some people are under the false impression that all cardio work is done slowly (at low to moderate levels of intensity) and for long durations up to an hour or more. This is not true. There's a wide range of intensity and duration that you can adjust to suit your needs. You should design a cardio routine to fit your goals and personal enjoyment. Try a higher intensity interval workout for 30 minutes and then you'll see the light.

When it comes to information and nutrition or cardiovascular exercise, I believe in a conservative approach. Most of the anti-cardio information (and nutritional quackery) is written by lay experts with no formal training. Some use their own worthless non-accredited certification (that they devised) as their main credential! The overwhelming opinion by the real experts in academia, medical and sports research, doctors and fitness experts (who have actually been university educated in the field) is that cardio work is important and should be done by all who are able to do it.

I would much rather trust people like Dr. Ken Cooper than the anti-cardio crown. For every single lay expert that's anti cardio, you could easily find many true professionals in medicine, research and academic who strongly think otherwise. Until these numbers are greatly changed, I strongly recommend that you keep doing your cardio work.

It's the same with stretching. There's a difference between injury-prevention stretching versus increasing-flexibility stretching. Before a strength-training workout, we do injury-prevention stretching for a few minutes. This is a minimal series of 20-second static-hold stretches. This series of stretches is done after the primary warmup. The primary warmup is 5 minutes of a cardio-type exercise like the Stairmaster, to elevate the core body temperature.

The best time to stretch is after you've preheated your muscles, like I just described. To increase your flexibility, you should make it a habit to devote about 10-15 minutes to doing stretches right after every cardiovascular workout. Be sure to first finish your very important 5-minute cooldown before you stretch. After the cooldown is complete, and you're still sweating, you should do your stretches while your muscles are still warm.

Q. *If I get very strong on the pullover machine, will this strength gain translate to improved chinning ability? Generally speaking, how does machine strength translate to free-weights exercises?*

A. The only guaranteed way to increase the ability to demonstrate strength in a particular movement is to perform that specific movement. If you want to improve your chinning ability, you must keep working on your chins. A gravitron machine, or doing assisted or weighted chins, would also be beneficial.

Exercises that are similar in movement, or work the same muscle groups, are beneficial and could assist you to get stronger in the chinning movement, if you keep chinning too. Motor learning is specific and exact. You must continue to work hard on the exact movement that you're trying to improve. There's no exact translation between free-weights exercises and machine exercises. There's also no exact formula to translate strength between any exercises, be they free-weights or machine.

Both free-weights and machines will make you stronger, but you must keep doing whatever the unit of strength measurement is. It goes both ways. If you exclusively do just the Hammer Chest Press or the Horizontal Tru-Press for years, you'll need an adjustment period when you go back to the barbell bench press. A lot of this is motor learning and just getting comfortable with the technique a gain. The same holds true with a person who only trains with barbells changes to machines, it will take a period of adjustment. A great example of this is the Tru-Squat. I don't care how much you can barbell squat, you'll have a hard time with a lot less weight (probably close to a third to half less), when you do the Tru-Squat for the first time.

I can only tell you what I believe in, so some may disagree with me. I'm not a big believer in long build-up cycles. First of all, if you're truly training for powerlifting, then you should already be lifting in a fairly low rep range. IF you're not, you should be. Most of your sets should be in the 3-6 rep range on a permanent basis as long as you're training for the purpose of powerlifting. Higher reps will not help you if your goal is to be a powerlifter.

It's no coincidence that long powerlifting build-up cycles and steroid usage usually co-exist. The long build-up cycle allows the lifter to cycle on and off drugs. It's the better of two evils, and at least better than staying on drugs all the time. The training cycle starts low as the steroid cycle begins. As the steroids kick in, so do the training cycle poundages. A natural lifter who's training with fairly low reps already on a permanent basis is not going to have months of build-up unless he's purely loafing and not training hard at all in the first half of the cycle (which is a waste of time).

Whenever I had a meet to prepare for, I would get a calendar and backdate my workouts from the meet to the present day. I would adjust my training a few months ahead of time so that my training schedule would be perfectly timed, and my last workout would be about four days before the meet. You would be surprised how some people just give no thought to this, and just keep training until the last minute and then realize that they are off schedule and will either have to compete with too little or too much rest, because they never backdated their training.

I always trained with low reps when competing, so a long buildup

223

was not needed, but I'd do a lot more doubles and singles in the last six weeks before the meet.

Q. *Because you were in the military, you probably have experience of shift working, and varying sleep patterns. What tips can you provide for shift workers, to help them sleep better and satisfy their sleeping needs?*

A. I've worked every type of shift work there is, from 24-hour shifts, to midnight till 8 am, 4 to 12, and regular day shifts. When I was working as a firefighter in the Air Force, I usually worked 24 hours on and 24 hours off, with an extra day off called a "Kelley Day" once every two weeks. On this shift, from 0730 'til about 1700 hours I had a scheduled work day with chores and regular fire training to do. It was a lot of work and I couldn't sit around. But after 5 pm I usually had "down time," which meant I could do whatever I wanted, such as sleep or watch TV, but I still had to stay in the station and respond to any emergency 'til 0730 the next morning. I would frequently not get a good night's sleep.

I was in Germany at the height of the Cold War. When the Soviets had invaded Afghanistan, things were real tense. We were flying fully loaded 24 hours a day and would usually have to get up for an in-flight emergency at least once a night. Anything wrong with the plane, like a low oil pressure light on (which is usually not serious), we still had to respond to and stand by on the runway. Sometimes we would have several of these emergencies, and we would be exhausted the net day.

You can adjust to any individual shift and get used to it, but the worst type of shift work is the revolving type when they rotate you, e.g., two regular days, two "Swings" (4 pm 'til midnight), 2 "mids" (midnight 'til 8 am), and then a break for three days. I worked this type of schedule for a while and it was a killer. My body could never get used to it due to the constant changing.

Here are a few things that helped me: I would try to keep my eating patterns the same. If I worked all night I would still have a good breakfast before going to bed. I had to make my room cold and dark so it would feel as though it was night. I couldn't sleep with sunlight coming in the room, or if I was feeling warm and sweaty, especially in summer. I'd put the air conditioning way up, or open the windows in winter and pile on the blankets. I even stapled a dark green army blanket to the window frame, over the regular blind, to keep the room dark and fool my body into feeling like it was actually night (during the day). I would also need the room quiet—television, radio, etc., off. For me, if I was not hungry, and made the room quiet, cold and dark, I slept like a log no matter what shift I worked.

BOB WHELAN'S Q & A

September 2001

Q. *I've had elbow and shoulder injuries, and I have to be especially careful to warm up these joints very well, otherwise I hurt myself. What do you think is the best way to warm up these joints?*

A. With your history of injuries I would do a five-minute cardio warmup followed by a series of mild (not painful) static stretches. Be sure not to overstretch. After the general warmup work, and a light specific warmup set, I would recommend training exclusively on a very slow rep speed protocol such as 10/10 cadence, on a permanent basis. This way you'll get an additional built-in warmup in the first few reps you do, and greatly reduce the risk of further injury.

Q. *What experience do you have of trainees who have much more responsive lower bodies than upper, or vice versa, and how do you deal with this?*

A. I get trainees all the time who *claim* to have an unresponsive part of their body, but just because they say it, doesn't mean that it's true. I've never had this problem, with any client after he/she has trained with me for several months. I balance their routines and then proceed to work their butts off in all the major areas of the body. They get balanced muscular development for their efforts (or quit because they can't take it, and thus stay "unbalanced").

The vast majority of the time, the "unbalanced" trainee is not doing something right and it's usually related to not working hard enough over all the major areas of the body. They are ignoring major planes of motion in their programs. It's usually when I first talk to someone on the phone (or during the initial training consultation) that they have all sorts of complicated issues. Once we start training, however, I usually see that there's no complicated issue that properly-applied and hard work won't solve.

Most of the time, when people claim to have their legs lagging behind their upper body, it's because they don't squat. The other main reasons are because they either don't squat enough, don't squat properly, or don't work hard enough on the squat (and wimp out on their sets). They are usually doing leg extension and leg curls (only), and maybe the leg press, and that's it for their legs. It's no wonder they have puny legs! Another problem is if they do squat, they are not going down low enough and are just "cracking" their knees in a partial way, with lots of weight. I get guys all the time who claim to squat the world, but when they squat for me, with about 75% of their claimed weight, they crash to the floor like a broken elevator shaft when I make them go lower than cracked-knee (quarter-rep) depth.

Many guys just don't squat hard, and quit the set when it gets too tough. Many of my beginner trainees do this. It takes some people a while before they finally get it. Squats are tough! They are hard work., They are supposed to be hard! If they are not brutal, you're doing something wrong—you're loafing and don't deserve results because you're not willing to work for them.

If you have a medical reason that prohibits you from squatting, make sure that you use a *good* leg press, like one from Hammer Strength or MedX. Most leg presses at commercial gyms are junk. Be sure to do trap bar deadlifts too, if possible, once per week.

A very common upper-body problem is that the pulling muscles are out of whack. Most guys spend a lot of time on their backs doing bench presses, but don't do nearly enough horizontal pushing. Most trainees do too many overall pushing exercises, and not enough pulling ones. My friend Jamie LaBelle, of The Quality Repetition in New York, has the same opinion about this. He even gives his new clients a three-to-one ratio of pulling to pushing exercises when they first sign up with him, due to the common imbalance of pushing and pulling for the upper body. After several months of this three-to-one ratio (and their strength is more balanced), then they can move into a more equally balanced routine. This is a good temporary way to get a problem corrected.

I generally try to make sure that the various planes of motion (horizontal and vertical) are equally covered by pushing and pulling exercises. Very rarely do you find that someone has the reverse imbalance. Guys hardly ever have over-developed pulling and under-developed pushing. This is mainly due to the ego connection with the bench press.

They key to results, no matter what part of the body, is regularly applied hard work. Most people are far too easy on themselves and don't work nearly as hard as they think.

Q. *Why do some trainers recommend increases in training volume as one advances, as opposed to paring down volume to a minimum?*

A. I don't know. Why do some trainers recommend anything and everything? There are many foolish trainers out there. This question could be reversed, as I'm sure there are many trainers who recommend the opposite. I think the question should be about what I recommend, not why others recommend something. I can't be boxed into a question that someone else gave his opinion on without knowing anything about the individual being trained.

Training volume depends on many things. What are your goals for the training? How old are you? How is your health? What's your injury history? How much time do you have to train? How long have you been training? What's your current strength level? Do you really enjoy training? What equipment do you have access to?

Once these questions have been answered, I can accurately devise a plan of action. Generally, if someone loves training, has a definite training-related goal, is young, tough, healthy and has access to (and is eager to use) a wide variety of equipment, then more volume is appropriate. It's very rare, in my opinion, that people fail to get results because of too much volume. Training frequency is much more of a problem than volume. Many guys go to the gym too many times per week. That's frequency. Volume is what they do after they get there. Many seem to spend 45 minutes just bench pressing, with nine other guys, don't even break a sweat, and spend more time looking in the mirror and going to the water fountain than they do training.

A common problem I see is the opposite of too much volume. Many people are making their workouts too abbreviated. They have good intentions, but are simply not doing enough work.

Q. *Would you recommend 20-rep squatting and 20-rep deadlifting in the same program, albeit on different days each week, or would you advise just one of them in any given program?*

A. There's nothing wrong with doing 20 reps on both the squat and deadlift in the same program. But it sure is brutally tough! It really depends on the person. I personally usually do slightly slower reps in the deadlift than the squat. I usually do no more than 12-15 reps for a high-rep deadlift set. I feel that form is especially critical in the deadlift, and as fatigue sets in people get sloppy with form, especially after 15 reps, and they get nicked. Minor back injuries are common in the deadlift after 15 reps, in my opinion. Although usually minor, they are still enough to affect your training in a negative way for a few weeks.

After about 15 reps on the deadlift, many trainees do just about anything to get the weight up, and the injury rate is higher due to body movement—twisting, jerking, shaking, not keeping the back flat, forgetting to thrust in the hips, etc. In my experience, the injury rate is higher after 15 reps of deadlifts, so that's usually as high as we go. Most of the time we don't even do 15. That's just the high end. We usually do 12 *heavy* reps in perfect form for more people who are not powerlifting. In my experience and opinion, I don't see this same effect concerning injury after 15 reps of the squat, so I sometimes use higher reps there.

Q. *How do you advise specialization on specific exercises, e.g., the overhead press?*

A. I don't advise people to specialize on specific exercises. I advise them to think of exercises as movements and planes of motion. I try to de-emphasize the ego connection with specific lifts, and focus on getting the whole body equally strong from all angles, not just in certain exercises (perhaps brag to your friends about).

If I have someone who wants to specialize on the military press, that's fine with me and all just in his own head. It's got nothing to do with me and won't affect how I train him at all. I'll work him hard when he does his military press, but will give that exercise no more special attention than any other major movement. He'll be worked equally hard in his chins or pulldowns, benches and rows, and squats and deadlifts. Thinking of planes of motion, or the function of muscles, also opens up a whole new world of training for you. You can now fill the void with many pieces of equipment—either machines or barbells. If you travel, no problem. Find the equipment to fill the functional need. It doesn't have to be any specific exercise. Horizontal push could be bench press, dumbbell bench press, Hammer bench press, Horizontal Tru-Press, Nautilus bench press, etc.

I've written repeatedly about not putting special attention on any one lift, especially the bench press. I've never bashed the bench press and never said not to do it—just don't get carried away with it. Don't give it special status over other major lifts. One pet peeve with me is the up-and-down view of the bench press by some muscle writers. It goes from being the king of upper-body exercises for some, to being based lately by some writers (often because they are not good benchers). There's one well known writer who used to be a big advocate of the bench press, but because he hurt his shoulder and can't bench press heavily anymore, now does not advocate the exercise. The bench press has more ego connection than any other lift, and causes problems for trainees who get ego addicted to it.

The same ego connection also affects writers who are not good at the bench press, (or who can no longer do it) and is the real reason why they don't recommend the exercise. The bench press is no more important than rowing, chins, squats, etc. *But* it's no less important either! Don't bash the bench press just because you're not good at it. Work at it just like any other major movement. It's not the "king" exercise that some think it is, but it's still an important exercise. It should not be de-emphasized any more than it should be overly emphasized. It's a major movement and one of the best exercises to use in the horizontal push.

If someone is competing in a strength sport, and that's the primary reason for training, then the routine will revolve more around the movements that will be used in the strength competition. Of course we'll spend more time on low-rep benching, squatting and deadlifting if someone is a competitive powerlifter. But we'll still do a complete and balanced routine from all the planes of motion after the primary competition lifts are done.

If someone is coming back from an injury, and has to catch up, we would specialize on the area of rehabilitation. I've had clients who have to rehab a certain area of the body. We train the rest of the body in a normal fashion and then do a rehab workout on just the area that needs rehab. The whole body is still worked. If a shoulder is being rehabbed, we still work the good shoulder with the isolateral machines in a normal fashion. After all the other work is done, we do rehab in is machines in a slow speed for the rehab area. This is one way that I may specialize on a certain body part. Also, if someone is severely imbalanced in strength and development, we may go to a Jamie LaBelle type three-pull-to-one-push plan, as explained earlier.

The key thing to remember is to think of your body as a unit. Make it strong from as many angles and planes as possible. Don't have an ego connection to certain lifts, but put equal emphasis on all the major movements that work the body in a balanced fashion. Don't be like the out-of-shape powerlifter who is strong in only three movements; and don't complain about things you're not good at either—work on them instead.

BOB WHELAN'S Q & A

November 2001

Q. *I'm in my early 40s. I reached the 300 bench press, 400 squat and 500 deadlift in my late 20s. Since then I keep injuring myself and can't reach those weights again. How can I rebuild my strength without injuring myself?*

A. My first advice would be to forget about those numbers. You're probably not competing in powerlifting if you've not been able to reach those numbers for over ten years. What's the hang up with those particular numbers? You should focus on building strength, not on demonstrating strength in a specific unit of measurement that obviously is damaging to your body. Demonstrate your strength in another mode or method that's safer for you. Try using some Hammer Strength or Southern Xercise units. Try training using a slow speed. You'd still be training for strength. You'd still be building strength. You should still lift as heavy as possible. You can still demonstrate your strength, but you need to *change the unit of measurement*. Those three particular lifts are not the end all to show the world how strong you are! Many powerlifters can't chin themselves once and are not tremendously strong when outside their three specific lifts. Just focus on getting strong.

Most people who train regularly (but who don't get injured) can continue to build strength well into their 40s and beyond. If you've been training regularly for all these years, and are not just coming back from one layoff after another, then your injuries should tell you something. Try training using a 10/10 speed. Cut down your poundages to about 60% and get 2 sets of 5 reps before you're entitled to increase the weight. Keep the repetition transition between positive and negative phases in a slow smooth motion with no fast jumps. Try this for a whole workout and see if it's for wimps! And if you're not suffering from just a form problem, try switching to the machines I mentioned previously, to substitute for the barbell exercises that are causing you problems.

233

~~

Q. *I've been using the Hammer Strength Deadlift. I've noticed in* *your past articles that both one-legged and two-legged deadlifts on* *this machine are performed with the back towards the plates as* *opposed to facing the plates. But I've been performing the deadlift* *facing the plate end of the machine. Can both variations of the* *exercise be performed either facing towards or away from the* *machine? Also, has anyone ever devised a rough rule-of-thumb for* *comparing the amount of weight lifted using the machine to that* *lifted using a barbell?*

A. There's *only one way* the machine is made to do the one-legged deadlift. So there's not much to talk about here. The foot of the non-lifting leg is placed on the rack made for it in back of the machine. There's nowhere else to put it. Here's the technique: Use the bottom handles (the top handles are for shrugs). Put the foot of the working leg in the middle of the platform and about an inch or so back from the front edge. You may have to adjust this a little, as it depends on your size. Put the foot of the non-working leg on the foot holder that's on the machine in the back. Grab the bottom handles while keeping the front knee bent. You must bend *well* over. Pull up to the standing position with your hands by your side. If your hands are out in front of you when you're standing upright with the handles, you must shift your feet and hand placement a little. Try to get 12 reps with each leg. If the weight is right, it should be *hard.* The one-legged deadlift is, however, only to be done on a Hammer Strength Deadlift machine—*never with a* *barbell.*

The regular two-legged deadlift can be performed either way around, but the machine is officially made to be used facing outwards in the same position as the one-legged deadlift. The grip is made for this too, as it's hard to hold onto the handles in the reverse position.

I started using the Hammer Deadlift at Drew Israel's house and he used it in the conventional Hammer Strength recommended way, so when I got my own I kept that same style. There are, however, some who believe that the reverse style is better and safer, including Dr. Ken. I asked Ken about this and here's his reply:

> [Regarding the two-legged/regular Hammer Strength Deadlift] "It is my opinion, one I've strongly expressed numerous times to Gary [Jones—son of Arthur] that while the handles are made to accommodate one facing *away* from the machine, I feel the strength curve is more appropriate, and feels better and safer, facing *into* the machine, even though it puts the hands/grip at somewhat of a disadvantage."

Regarding comparing the amount of weight lifted using the machine to the poundage lifted using a barbell, there's no exact translation between free-weight exercises and machine exercises. There's also no exact formula to translate strength between any exercises, be they free weights or machine. Free weights and machines both will make you stronger, but you must keep doing whatever the unit of strength measurement is.

The only guaranteed way to increase the ability to demonstrate strength in a particular movement is to perform that specific movement. If you want to improve your (barbell) deadlifting ability, you must keep working on your (barbell) deadlifts.

Exercises that are similar in movement, or work the same muscle groups, are beneficial and could assist you to get stronger. The Hammer Deadlift can assist you to get stronger in the barbell deadlift if you keep barbell deadlifting too. Motor learning is specific and exact. You must continue to work hard on the exact movement you're trying to improve.

Q. *What do you think of routines where we're advised to train* three, four or more days per week?

A. I don't endorse split routines and believe that if you train hard, then two whole-body workouts in a 7-10 day period is optimal and all that you're physically able to do. But I also believe that it's possible for some individuals, usually those with superior genetic advantages, to get good results with a four-day split routine. This is only if the split is properly balanced in a push/pull (or upper-body/lower-body) format with no muscle overlap. Though a minority of lifters may be able to train four days per week, I believe they would get better results by training their full body twice every 7-10 days. Forget about anything more than four days per week as it will not work without drugs. You might make short-term gains if you're young, but long-term will always lead to overtraining and/or injuries.

Regarding three *whole*-body workouts per week, many people who should know better are still fooled into thinking that more training frequency is better. They try to train doing three *whole*-body workouts per week. This is a mistake and too much if you're training in a high-intensity heavy and *hard* fashion.

When I say *hard*, I mean sets to failure with heavy weights, minimum rest between sets, compound exercises, balanced, whole-body higher volume training. Training *heavy* is not always the same as training *hard*. Many powerlifters train heavy but never even break a sweat. If you do a sub-maximum single and rest five minutes and then do another sub-maximum single, that isn't hard training. It may be heavy training, but not *hard*.

Another consideration is the type of routine you're using. *If you use a *very* abbreviated routine (usually unbalanced with just three or four exercises), but lift heavy and take a *lot* of rest, you may get away with training it three days a week. *If you train like we do at Whelan Strength Training—with a balanced, higher-volume, heavy-sets-to-failure (or beyond) routine—you're *physically*

236

unable to train more than twice per week.

If you truly train *hard* as I described above, cut down your whole-body workouts to no more than twice every week, and you'll feel a lot stronger and recovered for your training. Many so-called training fitness guidelines that recommend whole-body routines three times a week are just for general fitness and are mere toning routines. They are not meant for serious, hard strength training. If you train seriously, progressively and hard in a true high-intensity fashion, then you would be far better off training with fewer than three whole body sessions per week. (Once again, the WST guideline is *two* full-body workouts every 7-10 days.)

Q. *What experience of arm wrestling do you have? How would you recommend that someone train for arm wrestling?*

A. I've no experience in arm wrestling and, frankly, I've no interest in it, or desire to do it. No offense to the questioner personally, but generally speaking I usually associate arm wrestling with "low lifes" trying to show how strong they are, often in a bar room setting. (Of course, there are arm wrestlers who are very different characters and nice guys too.) There's a lot of technique in arm wrestling, and it does little to really show how strong you are. (I would personally like to see the bar-room arm wrestler in the gym with a bar on his back squatting, to see how strong he really is.)

I personally don't like the way subjects like arm wrestling, so called strength "feats" and "stunts", fitness fads, LIGHT Kettle Bell training, body weight exercise, Indian Clubs, grip ONLY trainees etc. have infiltrated their way into some of the STRENGTH training magazines and websites. I want traditional strength training info and not much else.

I'm not one to give advice for arm wrestling other than to train your whole body in a balanced fashion as I've previously explained. I would also recommend a lot of extra grip and forearm work. I would then contact Roger LaPointe at AtomicAthletic.com.

237

They make some special equipment for arm wrestling training. And join an arm wrestling organization and talk to some prominent arm wrestlers for arm wrestling advice.

Q. *What's your opinion on working your abs by kneeling on the* floor and placing a device on wheels on the floor in front of you, grasping it to support your upper body, then rolling forward to extend your body, then returning to starting position? Is this a safe and effective way to train abs? *I've seen a number of ads on TV for* different variations of this ab wheel.

A. This device will work your abs, though I've heard reports from some people that it can produce lower-back problems.

I prefer to work my abs in a strength-training fashion with progressive poundage increases, usually twice per week. Some people train abs several days per week (and you can probably get away with it if you're using the wheel and other non-progressive-poundage training devices).

It's the poundage that causes the micro trauma that requires the extra recovery, so if you strength train your abs with poundage increases, you should train your abs just like any other muscle—hard and relatively infrequently.

At WST we're doing 3/4 depth situps on a crunch board while holding a dumbbell on our chests. I'm up to 20 reps with a 90-pound dumbbell done just twice per week. You have to start light and slowly work up the poundage.

Q. *Do you recommend using a cambered bar for squats?*

A. To each his own, as I know many who swear by a cambered bar. I *personally* don't like it. Why? Just a matter of comfort I guess. I spent over thirty years using a regular Olympic bar and even have a permanent groove for it in my upper traps. Seriously!

I bought a cambered squat bar several years ago. While it's a great sturdy bar, I just prefer *the feel* of a regular Olympic bar. You have to try both and make up your own mind. Use less weight at first with the cambered bar because the weight is shifted slightly differently than on a regular bar, and that slight shift can cause an injury if you're not used to it. For your first few workouts, following several light warmup sets, perform your work sets considerably lighter than you used to with the straight bar, to get the feel of the exercise before going heavy.

BOB WHELAN'S Q & A

January 2002

Q. *How should a competing athlete such as a basketball player train with weights in-season?*

A. A basketball player, and any other type of athlete, should continue to strength train during the actual competitive season. You shouldn't be at your strongest and most physical ready state *before* the season. You should continue to get stronger as the season develops. While the questioner in that issue, and the one in this one, come from different sporting backgrounds, the answers to both are the same.

Q. *How often do you use thick-handled bars at Whelan Strength Training?*

A. For several years I used thick handles regularly, even on my machines. I used mostly 2-inch handles, but used the 3-inch bar for benches and a 2.5-inch bar for military presses. A few years ago I got my bench press up to 380 with a pause, with the 3-inch bar. My military press was up to about 220 x 6 with the 2.5. I loved using the thick bars but began to develop elbow problems. I finally figured out why—the 3-inch bar. It was painful for me to admit this to myself, as I'd been a big thick-bar advocate for years. I went back to regular handles for pushing, and my elbows are fine now.

This caused me to reevaluate the benefits of using thick bars for pushing movements. They do little for the grip when pushing, but mainly just look cool to use. They don't really make you stronger than regular handles and bars do, as when I switched back to a regular bar I had to start a little lighter because I wasn't used to the thinner handle. The thinner handle actually felt harder for a while.

I believe that you'll adapt to the 2-inch handles/bars for pushing movement and these are actually more comfortable once you adjust. You may also like using them just because they look cool, but they are not any harder to use for pushing than the thinner handles. It's only for pulling movements that the thick bars/handles are beneficial and more difficult. The 3-inch bar is never comfortable, however, and turns the bench press into an odd-object movement.

I still use thick bars at WST, but mostly only use the 2-inch bar/handles for pulling movements. The 2.5-inch and 3-inch bars have cobwebs on them.

Q. *Please tell me what I can do in conjunction with regular workouts to train my rotator cuffs. They don't hurt, and I've no prior injuries; I'm just trying to be smart and safe so that I don't regret, someday after I've hurt myself, that I hadn't trained them.*

A. I personally don't feel that extra work is needed for most people. I would only use it for rehab and for people such as baseball pitchers who frequently injure this area. You could add a set of the L-fly two times a week after your workouts, increasing the resistance gradually over time. The rotator cuff muscles only serve to stabilize the shoulder joint, and don't have a big potential for strength gains. Be careful to do the L-fly slowly, with reps above 12.

I've never done the L-fly myself, and hardly ever get injured. Just warm up thoroughly, use weights you can handle properly, use good form, and most people shouldn't have rotator cuff problems. Regular compound pulling movements should work the rotator cuff just fine for most people.

Q. *I dropped flies from my pec work to concentrate on the big chest exercises (bench and dips().* However, my pecs don't look as *full as when I was using flies. Should I reintroduce one set of flyes, and make sure that I can still recover, or stay only with the big chest exercises?*

A. Keep doing the major movements like benches and dips and just add a couple of sets of flies if it makes you feel better. The addition of this little isolation exercise to your program (so long as it's not followed by other additions) won't hurt your recovery.

Q. *What's your opinion of pullovers? What safety considerations are there when performing this exercise at home with a barbell? Is it considered a puling or pushing exercise, and which muscles does it target?*

A. Pullovers are a great exercise. They are a lot safer when done on a good machine (e.g., Hammer), but can still be effective with a barbell or dumbbell for some people.

For years I used to do pullovers with an ez-curl bar. I would lay on a bench and take a very narrow grip and lower the weight to the floor and then pull it up over my face and onto my chest. You must start very light or it can mess up your shoulders by overstretching them. The exercise can really increase your flexibility in this area. It's a borderline dangerous exercise. I did it and like it, but that's because I was able to do the exercise. Some people can't. If pullovers hurt you, don't do them with a barbell. Try doing them light and see how your shoulders can take them, and if you're flexible enough to do them.

242

They also can mess up your face if you try one rep too many. I pulled "one too many" several times in the past, and got black eyes from them. Seriously! People thought I'd been in a fight when all I'd done was train. I'd turn my head sideways while doing the pullover, to miss my nose, but *drag* the bar over the side of my face. I was crazy (or crazier!) in my younger days.

Pullovers work both the upper-body pushing and pulling muscles, but I put them in the pulling category overall. One reason why some people called the pullover "the upper-body squat" is because it works almost every muscle in your upper body. Even your abs get worked on the Hammer machine which I have now.

Q. *I've a cocky student who wants me to give him a "brutally hard" workout. He's heard about me training other students, and that I train them hard 2-3 times a week, and that they are sore on their off days. He says that no workout has ever been hard for him, and he's challenged me to try to make him sore. Should I immediately give him what he says he wants, or work him progressively like I do the other students I train?*

A. My philosophy has always been that as long as a client has the proper attitude—i.e., listens, shows respect and puts his trust in you to train him—then it's your duty to train him as hard as he's able to tolerate safely, but never to purposely waste him.

But in this case, since he challenged you, and so long as he uses good form, is young and there's no fear of injury or harm, it sounds like he's fair game to me, as he's in need of an attitude adjustment. But this sort of approach is absolutely out of the question for older people or anyone who isn't tough, in very good condition, and really up for it.

I've had young, healthy and fit guys come in with attitudes for the orientation session, and they don't pay any attention. In these cases I stop the orientation and tell them we'll have a workout first. Then they listen.

Q. *Do you incorporate any negative-only training into your programs? Art Jones was a proponent of this, but I never hear much about it from anyone else. I for one use it with my female trainees on machine movements, and they respond very well. But it's hard to use with my male clients because I can't spot safely due to the high loads. The only real drawback is that soreness can be extreme, and it's hard to recover from.*

A. I'm not knocking it, but I don't use negative-*only* training, and never have. I know a number of people use it and like it, and that's great. Personally, I just don't see the reasoning to *not do* the concentric part of the movement.

Q. *Will you be posting any more letters from the late Charles Smith on Natural Strength.com, or is what's up there now all there is?*

A. Dennis Weis was kind enough to lend me his entire collection. Stuart had the collection previously and was putting them in *Hardgainer* several years ago. I think I probably stopped posting them for the same reason Stuart did.

I had a lot more letters left, but after reading them I figured that what was already on the website was the basic information you could get form them. Chas was entertaining, but there was a lot of gossip and innuendo type stuff, and a lot of the same material is repeated.

The strength field has a lot of interesting behind-the-scenes information that Chas brought out, but you have to balance that info. There's the possibility that Chas could have been an angry, bitter old guy too. (Vic Boff doesn't agree with a lot of what Chas said, particularly about Jowett.) I think it's a mixture of the two—some good behind-the-scenes info, and Chas being angry and bitter. You have to read a lot between the lines and not take everything he says at face value.

Q. *I've always been told to do abs without weight for hundreds of reps. I was wondering if I should start to train my abs with weights.*

A. I would work abs with two heavy workouts a week. At WST we do weighted crunches with an adjustable dumbbell. If you use an incline board, be careful not to go back too far with a dumbbell on your chest, or you could strain your lower back. Start going about halfway down and slowly work to about three-quarters depth. Keep reps under 20, and keep adding weight.

Q. *Do you train any competitive powerlifters or athletes, and how much do they lift? Who's the strongest person you've trained?*

A. When you get paid to train people, you get a lot of a short-term people who just want a jump start. Some just want some motivation or advice, and a few workouts. I've had some top-level powerlifters come in over the years on a short-term basis, including a few world champion drug-free lifters; but I'm not going to take any credit for their success by bragging that I trained them. I get a lot of visitors to WST, and I also get a lot of short-term and even singe-workout clients.

On a long-term basis, I don't have any powerlifting clients now, and few overall. Paying me by the hour is not as financially efficient for powerlifting training because powerlifters usually take a lot of rest between sets. After they get some short-term advice and training they can go train on their own for free, and take all the time they want between sets. Some of the powerlifters I've trained over the short term were not too impressive in strength outside the three lifts they compete in, and I don't think they enjoyed the experience training with me because their overall conditioning wasn't good. WST isn't a fun short-term place—you have to get used to it over time, as your conditioning progresses.

I think the whole athlete thing is greatly overrated. I train some lawyers who are stronger, more motivated and train harder than most of the athletes. For some reason, people are more impressed when you train guys who play games. In the gym, the games they play makes no difference. A lot of lawyers and accountants are ex-jocks who miss the competition and training. They want to train! A lot of the athletes don't like training and are just training because they feel they have to. A lot of trainers/coaches are just feeding their childhood fantasies of playing pro sports. Athletes usually don't train any harder than the regular Joe who comes in. I train human beings regardless of their profession.

I've been in business since 1990. I've met many people who were real strong in some lifts but who are not athletes, not famous, and unknown. Some of the clients with the best improvements are still not what most people would consider strong, because they started at such a very low level to begin with. I don't like to tell the story only with numbers, as they can be misleading. /many of the greatest success stories are not done justice by numbers.

Q. *Most of the old-timers from the twentieth century don't seem to have used odd objects. Does the mass production of the barbell,*

starting with the Milo Barbell Company in the early 1900s, have something to do with it?

A. From the early 1900s 'til the early 1990s, odd-object lifting was only rarely done, as a test of strength. It's a fact, however, that many cultures have used odd objects, mainly stones, for thousands of years. Bob Hoffman and others had positive things to say about some of the old, old, old-timers, many of whom performed feats of strength with odd objects, but most of this was in a past tense way and they were usually just feats of strength (not training), especially after about 1910.

The point is that after the mass production of the barbell started, there was very little information advocating the use of odd objects in the traditional Iron Game literature. There have always been obscure cultures that used odd objects as far back as recorded history, but most Iron Gamers didn't even consider odd objects as training tools. From around the early 1990s there was, however, a new lease of life for them in very limited circles.

As far as commercialism being the reason, no one except the fanatical fringe lifted weights prior to the start of the fitness craze, around the 1970s. Now, training and fitness are mainstream. Odd objects for training were nowhere to be found from about 1910 to 1990, and this had nothing to do with commercialism. It had to do with progress. Using odd objects today for the core of your training (not finishers) is like going back to the horse and buggy after the car was invented. Odd objects are a fun way to test strength and can be used as finishers, but only by the able bodied. To be used as the core of actual training, odd objects are clearly inferior to the barbell, which is why they were rarely used by the old-timers after the invention of the adjustable barbell.

Q. *Which exercise stimulates your metabolism/physiology the*

most?

A. In my opinion, in order, starting from the hardest: high-rep squat, Hammer Strength One-Legged Deadlift, regular deadlift. This answer is very subjective, but in my opinion nothing beats the high-rep squat (usually 20 reps) for overall metabolic stimulation. It works the largest muscles in your body and it takes everything you've got to get 20 or more reps with a challenging weight. The one-legged deadlift used on a Hammer Strength deadlift machine is also a very difficult exercise and most of my clients dread this one *more* than the regular two-legged deadlift. The regular two-legged deadlift would be number three on my list of exercises that provide the most metabolic stimulation, with the good leg presses such as Hammer and MedX fourth. They are all exercises that work the largest muscle groups of the body, but the order is subjective and a matter of opinion.

Vic Boff

On November 3, 2001, at the Fifth Capital City Strength Clinic, Vic Boff was honored and awarded the first Physical Culture Award. It will be called "The Vic Boff Physical Culture Award" in the future, and given at each Capital City Strength Clinic.

Vic is one of the most vocal critics of steroid use in the Iron Game. He's written several books and hundreds of articles on natural strength training and health living. He owned several health food stores in the 1960s, was a good all-around athlete, a competitive boxer and triple-A minor league baseball player. HE was also a champion wrist wrestler and long-time member of The Polar Bear Club. He was close friends with John Grimek, Sig Klein and George Jowett. He's the founder of The Oldtime Barbell & Strongman Association, and has been its president for over twenty years, keeping the traditions alive by honoring the great leaders of the Iron Game. It's about time that Vic was honored. Good job, Vic, and as you say... *"Carry on."*

248

BOB WHELAN'S Q & A

March 2002

Q. *A physical therapist recently commented that my farmer's walk will lead to bad rotator cuffs due to the vibratory type action of the weight as I walk down my gravel driveway (about 150 feet long). Do you agree?*

A. No. It sounds like you have a non-lifting physical therapist. Any exercise could bother some people for various reasons, but to make a general statement like that of the therapist's, is comparable to saying that squats will hurt your knees, or deadlifts will hurt your back. The problem with many medical personnel—doctors, registered nurses, therapists of all types, etc.—is that they have a good *general* knowledge about the anatomy and various conditions of the body, but lack the specific knowledge that would enable them to apply what they know to strength training. The therapist may know quite a bit about the body's general physiological response to exercise, what happens to the body when it gets injured, and *general* information on exercise rehab, but has a poor or non-existent strength-training background.

If your doctor or therapist tells you not to lift instead of explaining how you *can* lift, I'd look for a new doctor or therapist. Interview or investigate to find yourself a doctor/therapist who strength trains him/herself.

Unless you've some sort of genetic shoulder problem, or have a previous injury that causes the farmer's walk to bother your rotator cuff/shoulder area, I'd continue with the farmer's walk. It's a good exercise and should help to strengthen your traps, upper back, grip and shoulders.

249

Q. *If you had to condense everything you know into five simple training principles, what would they be?*

1. Good mental focus

Think positively, but not just a passive positive attitude. That won't work. You should have a little hostility when training, just as football players and other athletes do during a game. Athletes may temporarily hate and despise their opponents during a game. You should have that same attitude towards the barbells and equipment during your workouts. Attack the equipment as if it has just attacked your family, like a mother bear whose cubs are threatened. Train like you're ready for war and your life depends on it.

Very importantly, learn to enjoy training even though it's brutally hard. Good examples of this are marathon runners. They usually love to run, and get runners' high from it even though it's brutally tough. Running a marathon is extremely tough and painful, but marathon runners usually love doing it or they wouldn't be able to take it. I've been annoyed by some writers who scoff at being able to enjoy training. They just don't get it. They act as though training is some sort of negative act of suffering through pain. Not true at all. Work brutally hard, but still *enjoy* it, just as marathon runners enjoy running.

Another bit of advice about mental focus, and a pet peeve of mine, is lazy advice given by some writers about talking during workouts. The usual advice is: *Don't talk during workouts*. This is only realistic if you train alone. If you train in public or with a training partner or coach, you *must* and *will* talk. After a brief conversation during a planned resting period, be sure to take about 20 seconds in order to re-focus. Only then, after you've refocused, should you begin your next set. Never just go straight from talking to lifting, or you're doomed to fail.

2. Good form

Or, as Jamie LaBelle coins it, "The Quality Repetition." Stick to the rules of protocol of whatever style you're using. The rules are a little different depending on the rep speed that you use, exercise selection, the purpose of your training, and whether you use barbells or machines.

You shouldn't cut corners and get sloppy just to get one more rep. Avid body twisting and heaving. Stay balanced. Make each rep a deliberate and controlled effort, and don't allow the rest to degenerate into a blur of uncontrolled effort where each rep is indistinguishable from the next. Pause for a second at the mid-point of most pulling movements (*between* the positive and negative phases). Lower the weight slowly for at least 4 seconds even on regular-speed movements.

3. Progression

This is the key to muscular size and strength no matter what type of strength training you do. As George Jowett said, "Progression is the law of growth. Whoever accedes to that law will succeed." This is common sense, but forgotten by many, especially those who train using a controlled or slow speed. Even if you're training with slow rep, progression is still the key. Moving even slower a weight that's already too light, will not work. It must be as *heavy* as you an possible handle at the desired speed, to work.

There are two main theories of progression: (a) progression by performance, and (b) progression by time. I believe in, and usually use, progression by performance. Your performance dictates when you're ready to add weight. You have a rep goal for the set and when that goal is reached add weight.

Progression by time is when you have a planned schedule of when to add weight. You could add a pound a week, or 5 pounds every 2 weeks, or whatever your plan is. I don't use this method, but many do and get great results from it. To each his own, as both methods work depending on what style of training you're involved in, and your level of experience and development. As long as you're adding weight to the bar or machine on a regular basis, then you should reap the rewards of training.

Striving to add weight is the key. AS you advance through the years into the intermediate and advanced stages of your training, adding weight will not be as easy as it was when you were a beginner. This is common sense and only natural.

Many people get the wrong idea and think they had a bad workout if they didn't add weight on any exercise during a workout. This is a mistake. Judge your workouts by your true and honest *effort*. The truth is, as you advance, you may go for several workouts without adding weight. You can even go for extended periods. You may not be *ready* or physically able to add weight, especially as you advance to the advanced stages of ten or more years of training. Be patient. Work with your training weight, strive to hit the rep goal, but only judge your workout by your effort or otherwise you'll drive yourself crazy and develop a negative attitude which will hurt your training.

If you truly added weight at *every* workout—not counting false progression at the beginning of a training cycle, but true personal best increases—you could be the strongest man in the world fairly quickly.

Always have the *goal* to add weight. Always *strive* to add weight but never add weight before you're ready. Remember, judge your workouts by your honest and true effort. *Always striving* for progression is the key.

4. Balanced training program

A rule I follow is using an equal number of pushing and pulling exercises at each workout. I usually perform a pushing and a pulling exercises for the horizontal and vertical planes for the upper body at each workout, and rotate the leg press, deadlift and some type of squat (regular, front or Tru-Squat). This may, however, be too much for some people. Some respond better to training the horizontal and vertical plane just once a week each. For some advanced trainees I employ two leg movements in one workout, e.g., the Hammer Deadlift and Leg Press.

It's a good idea to alternate the pushing and pulling exercises so there's built-in recovery between exercises even though you're not actually resting. You'll lose too much strength if you do multiple pushing or pulling exercises back to back, e.g., overhead press followed by the bench press. I usually have my charges perform three exercises in a row with no rest between sets, and then have them take a minute or two off. If there's a leg exercise in the group—squat, leg press or deadlift—it will be put last in the group of three exercises. If there are two leg movements in the same workout, a longer rest between each group of exercises is allowed.

5. Recovery and nutrition

I get many people who claim that no matter what they do, they can't seem to gain any muscle. This is usually utter nonsense. The first question I ask is, "What did you have for breakfast today?" Incredibly, most either have a very small breakfast, or no breakfast at all. If you're trying to gain muscular weight, you *must* eat a big breakfast every day. (Of course, you must also train hard.) If you don't eat a big breakfast each day, then stop now and read no further, because you're wasting your time and are doomed to fail. I give an orientation to all my clients in which I teach them about various important topics before we even touch any equipment. One of the main things we cover is nutrition. No pills, powders or "magic" potion; instead, *food!*

Nutrition is about absorption, not just what you put down your throat. You can't get it all at just dinner, as otherwise most of the nutrition will be passed through without being absorbed. We already lose about 12 hours a day (between dinner and breakfast, approximately 6 pm to 6 am) of our potential nutrition intake time;

253

and this assumes that you *do* eat breakfast! If you don't eat breakfast, you may spend 18 of every 24 hours without consuming any nutrition. What law says that you must have cereal for breakfast? Why not chicken, vegetables, salad, potatoes, etc.?

Have you ever thought of setting your alarm clock for 2 am and getting up for an extra meal? Most regular people wouldn't dream of it, but a champion will.

For lunch, do you regularly eat sandwiches or do you eat a big knife-and-fork type meal? If you're trying to gain weight, it could make all the difference. A cafeteria-style knife-and-fork type meal with salad, vegetables, meat, fish or chicken, and rice or potatoes is far more beneficial for gaining weight than a simple sandwich-type lunch.

You also need 5-9 pieces of fruit and vegetables per day. It's hard to fill that bill with sandwiches. Use sandwiches as your snacks between meals.

Do you eat two cans of tuna packed in water per day in between your meals—not as meals, but between them? If you're dedicated and committed, you'll do it. You can also use chicken or turkey if you get sick of tuna. You should/could drink a *gallon* of skim milk per day. If you really need a lot of calories, drink a gallon of skim milk *and* eat two cans of tuna per day!

Don't waste your money on powders and amino acids. A gallon of milk per day will give you about 130 grams of protein, and 2 cans of tuna will give you around 90 grams. That's over 200 grams of protein *excluding* your threes.

Get enough sleep. This is the missing element in many training programs. Many young single guys I train have this problem at first. They claim to be doing everything right. They train hard, eat well and do cardio. Their problems are with alcohol use and sleep, which are frequently related. They go out drinking at bars and stay up too late too many nights per week. One weekend night a week will probably not hurt too much, but if you're carousing into the

254

wee hours of the morning two or more night per week, it's definitely going to hurt your progress—no doubt about it. The more nights per week that you do it, the more damaging it will be.

Be disciplined! Get your sleep or you'll pay with slow progress and wasted effort.

Q. *Do you use much training with slow reps at WST? What's your experience with slow reps in general?*

A. Over the years I've developed a lot of respect for slow training. It's a brutally tough form of training. At WST we use it periodically. We may use it for a few weeks or a few workouts, and then go back to regular speed. It's *excellent* for rehab. I have some rehab. I have some rehab and older clients—joint problems—who use it exclusively, and it works well. It's *safe* and almost impossible to get injured using it.

But don't let that give you the wrong idea. It really is *tough*. Many guys hate it because it's so tough, and some have even called in sick and gone home to bed after their first *slow* workout.

We've tried various, e.g., 8/8, 5/5, 5/5/5, 10/10 etc. IT mainly works well with machines, and can be dangerous with many barbell exercises. I have some clients who love it and I let them use it all the time. It's very popular with my women clients, almost all of them want to do slow training permanently.

Q. *After hearing stories of the machine, I thought I'd give the Tru-Squat a try, in my local gym. I followed the instructions on the machine, had it counterweighted with 25 pounds on the long arm, and I kept my feet underneath me. When I squatted down it irritated my knees similar to a hack squat. Did I do something*

wrong? Barbell squats don't irritate my knees.

A. I've had a Tru-Squat for several years. It works very well for most people, but I've had a few people who it always seemed to bother. They usually had a pre-existing condition that would be bothered to some degree by any sort of leg exercise. There's some technique involved here. The *official* recommendation of Southern Xercise is to stand straight up in an exact barbell squat position. I recommend to my clients to move their feet about an inch forward of straight up; *not too far,* just an inch or so. You may also be going down too far. This machine goes down very deep, well below parallel. Try putting the pin in the second hole up from the bottom and see how that feels. Finally, when you push up you should be driving *backwards* and upwards.

For most people, the Tru-Squat will usually not bother the knees if it's done properly. Unlike the hack squat and 45-degree leg presses the Tru-Squat allows for a great deal of hip extension if the hips keep in contact with the pad. People will have problems with the machine if they allow their hips and back to come off the pad, and if they don't concentrate on pushing through the heels.

Q. *What do you think of legal pro hormones?*

A. They should be avoided unless needed for a legitimate serious medical reason, and used under strict medical supervision. Just because something is legal doesn't make it good. Many steroids can also be obtained legally, with a prescription, from a crooked doctor. Despite the phony claims by the manufacturers of the pro hormones, they are no natural and frequently have harmful side effects.

Q. *Do you insist that your clients perform a "cool down" after* training? If so, what precisely do you have them do?

A. Yes, I insist that they do a five-minute cooldown, but not after their strength-training workouts they do with me. Cooldown is a cardiovascular term. I insist that my clients take a five-minute minimum cooldown after they do their cardio exercise, which they usually do on their own outside of WST.

Q. *I've had some serious trauma to the L5/S1 area of my lower back and can't* squat or stiff-legged deadlift anymore. I purchased a Tru-Squat machine, and the problem was solved for the squats. The problem is with my hamstrings. Leg curls have never seemed *to do the trick for my hamstrings. I've access to a glute and* hamstring apparatus *that looks like a modified back extension. I'm* wondering how it compares to a stiff-legged deadlift and hamstring curl.

A. I can't be sure without seeing it, but it sounds like it probably does work the same muscle group. It wouldn't work exactly the same as the stiff-legged deadlift, but would be close enough to serve as a good replacement exercise as long as it doesn't bother you.

I'd recommend you investigate the Hammer Strength Deadlift machine. Used properly, at least for most people, it's very safe. One- and two-legged versions of the deadlift can be performed on this machine. These two exercises work the glutes, hamstrings and lower back very effectively. I have people of all ages and conditions who can deadlift with the Hammer version but are unable to deadlift safely with a bar.

BOB WHELAN'S Q&A

May 2002

Q. *What kind of progression scheme do you prefer, and do you recommend a certain one to your clients?*

A. Nothing complicated—have a set/rep goal and add weight when you've reached it, usually 5 pounds, but it depends on the exercise. That's it. There are many ways to do it, but this is what I do.

Q. *How can I make an adjustable sandbag like the ones you use at WST?*

A. Go to an Army/Navy store or any military surplus store and buy duffel bags. Cut off the straps. Buy several smaller bags, too, each about the size of a pillowcase. Go get or buy some sand. Put 50 pounds of sand in each of the several smaller bags and 25 pounds of sand on one bag. This will allow you to progress in 25-pound increases rather than 50. Wrap the smaller bags completely in duct tape after having filled and tied them to keep them from spilling and breaking. There should be a few sizes of duffel bags to buy. I have one that holds up to about 225 pounds, and I have a huge bag that can hold up to about 325 pounds. Good luck!

Q. *What's your preferred exercise for developing size and strength in the forearms?*

A. Although just your regular training involving holding a heavy bar will build some strength in your forearms, there are many specific ways to build their strength. Here are some of the most common exercises that I've used: reverse curls (especially with a thick bar), using thick bars in your workout for pulling movements, wrist curls, timed bar hangs, plate pinch gripping, Titan's Telegraph Key (from IronMind), adjustable plate-loaded crusher grip machine (made by Jubinville or IronMind), Weaver stick or lever bar; and my favorite of all, the wrist roller. Be sure to use the wrist roller to work both sides of the forearms—palms up and palms down—or sets done with some reps focusing on extension and others on flexion.

Q. *Do you need to train to muscular failure to get maximum muscular and strength results? Do you always train to failure at WST?*

A. No, you don't have to train to muscular failure to get maximum results. Although I usually do train to failure, the primary stimulus for muscles strength and growth is poundage progression. As long as you're increasing the load, then you should get good results. We usually, but not always, train to failure at WST. It depends on the purpose or goal for the training.

Most of my clients are not powerlifters or competitive strength athletes. If you're a powerlifter, Olympic lifter, strongman competitor, or anyone who wants to be able to demonstrate strength in a one-rep max unit of measurement, then, at least some of the time, you must train like that unit of measurement. If you want to be able to demonstrate strength in that format, you must train for strength in a similar fashion and in the same energy system. Pyramid-type training working to very low reps would usually be the way to go for that type of goal. Several warm-up sets would be required to get a maximum or near-maximum double or single rep in training.

Since most athletes such as basketball, football, hockey, and baseball players don't need to demonstrate strength in a single or very low-rep fashion and don't even use a barbell in their chosen sport, then going to failure in a moderate rep range is a beneficial and safe way for them to train.

Training to failure is also time productive as it involves fewer warm-up sets and fewer work sets. One hard work set to muscular failure is usually all that's needed. The reward for your hard work is the need for fewer work sets to get the job done. It's great for the everyday working person who's training for health benefits but doesn't have a lot of time to spend in the gym. Athletes who are already tired and banged up with minor injuries from playing their sport will benefit greatly from the hard but brief strength work you get as a result of training to failure.

Training to failure is the most time efficient way to get maximum strength results. It's not necessarily the best way for everyone, but it offers the most bang for the training buck as far as time is concerned. My clients pay me by the hour, so training to failure is very beneficial for the vast majority of my clients. The goal and reason why you train will make either training to failure or not training to failure the right way to train *for you.*

For many years, when I was powerlifting, I didn't train to failure. I lifted as heavily as I could and got plenty of rest between sets. I also experimented with several schemes of working out such as using the pyramid-style of training for the competitive lifts, i.e., squat, bench press, and deadlift. I did the assistance exercises using a moderate rep range done at a faster pace to muscular failure.

A few of the powerlifters I've trained at WST have done it this way, too. They would just come to me part time, usually about once a week or so. They would get a good to-failure whole-body workout with me for their overall strength and conditioning. Since they were paying me by the hour, they would do their time-consuming primary competition lifts on their own because they are done slower with longer rest periods between sets (pyramid-style training). Use your imagination and you can devise several effective ways to train.

There are many individuals and organizations in the strength-training field who waste much time and energy arguing over pointless issues. Going to muscular failure is just one of these issues (along with rep speed, multiple or single sets, doing power cleans, use of odd objects, etc.).

You can go to muscular failure doing pushups and lifting light weights, and you'll get nowhere. If you train to failure, you must still put primary emphasis on poundage progression for it to be effective. Going to failure without poundage progression is no better than doing calisthenics. Training without going to failure will probably take longer timewise, but as long as you're adding weight to the bar, it will work just fine.

Poundage progression is the single element that unifies all successful strength-training programs regardless of organization, affiliation, or cult. Progression is the unifying factor that makes all strength-training methods work. Any of these methods can be the correct method for different individuals. The person using a given method probably has his own particular reason and goals that makes whatever method he chooses seem sensible to him.

Always remember that the main stimulus for muscular strength and size is *poundage progression*, not going to failure, tension, rep speed, equipment, etc. as far as the question "Should you train to muscular failure?" it all depends on the goal of your training and what you enjoy.

Q. *What are your thoughts on combining all pulling exercises in one workout and all the pushing exercises in another and alternating the two workouts according to the individual's recovery abilities?*

A. As long as you're getting your work done, are eating well, getting enough recovery, and are progressing in poundages doing the basic lifts, then a multitude of programs can work. A pull/push program worked for me when I was stationed at Spangdahlem Air Base in Germany years ago. I was a firefighter on 24-hour shifts. Because of my shift work I composed a push/pull style routine that served me very well. I trained a push day, then I had to work 24 hours, then I trained a pull day followed by another day of work. Each workout I did about three sets of 6-8 on noncompetitive lifts and worked the three powerlifts in a pyramid fashion with fairly low reps, as I was competing in powerlifting at the time. Sometimes the workout would be a lot shorter if I was tired or I would occasionally miss a day.

My push day was something like this: bench press, incline press, behind-neck press, triceps press, squat, leg press, leg extension. My pull day was something like that is: barbell pullover with ez-curl bar, cable pulldown, bent-over row, upright row, curl, good morning/deadlift (alternating), and sometimes the leg curl.

I was training in the sparsely equipped military gym at that time. Overall the equipment was basic, but the training atmosphere was great.

My training has evolved since then, and I do less volume now. I've also done something like push on Monday, pull on Tuesday, and whole body on Friday with good results, although I wouldn't recommend it for most people. If you enjoy training, get adequate recovery, and split your program properly in an upper body/lower body or push/pull format, it could be a productive way to train. I believe, however, that two whole-body workouts every 7-10 days works best for most natural lifters.

Q. *What program would you recommend for someone wanting to compete in strongman competitions?*

A. First, I'd check the organization that is sponsoring the event and make sure that it's a natural event, i.e., has mandatory drug testing and/or polygraph testing. Most strongman contests, even those that claim to have "random" drug testing, are a joke and filled with steroid users. Usually there's no real effort made to weed them out.

An organization that's 100% natural and which I recommend is Bill Clark's All-Round Weightlifting Association. Check it out at www. USAWA.com. find out which events are going to be in the competition, as many of them are free wheeling and you need time to practice them.

You need to practice doing the exact movements you're going to be doing in competition. Contact the organization and find some competitors who live near you to practice with. Buy videos of the events and be sure to watch an event before actually competing. Try to enter a novice meet first.

You may want to contact Roger LaPoint at Atomic Athletic and find out what equipment you may need to practice with. Roger sells most of the equipment used. (AtomicAthletic.com)

As far as strength training with conventional equipment, I'd work the whole body focusing on very low reps similar to a powerlifting workout. Without knowing the exact lifts in competition, I can't be specific on this. Just work your whole body with equal emphasis on pushing and pulling movements. Keep doing the major compounds—squat, deadlift, press, row, bench press, etc. work abs, neck, and grip, too, as always. The only change would be to do lower reps and go heavier in a pyramid-type format.

Q. *I travel a lot and don't always have access to weights. When weights aren't accessible, how can I get in a good maintenance workout using bodyweight exercises alone?*

A. If your goal is to maintain maximum levels of strength, you'll not be able to do it with bodyweight exercises alone. You'd just be delaying a sinking ship. To stop it from sinking, you must train with progression, which you don't get with bodyweight exercises unless you can tie weights to your body somehow. They are better than nothing, though, so if it's a choice between watching TV and doing the bodyweight exercises, then by all means do them.

It would be better to look in the Yellow Pages and find a good gym in the area and just pay the single workout rate. As a last resort, some good bodyweight exercises are pushups or dips between chairs, chins or pullups, situps, or crunches, and bodyweight squats done slowly. Better still, *find a gym.*

Q. *what methods to you use to get psyched up for a hard set? What other mental training techniques do you recommend?*

A. I like to have a time limit in my head. I say to myself, "This set is going to last less than one minute. I can go all out for just one minute." By having a time factor goal, it's a lot easier to get focused and go all out.

Sometimes it's good to learn to take the pressure off. This was especially important to me during my days of powerlifting competition. I would attack the weights with abandon because I would tell myself, "What's the worst thing that could happen? I just miss the lift! So what? I'm not going to die or anything!" This took the pressure off at critical times and helped a great deal.

Another pressure-reducing technique is always to think of only competing against yourself and not others. If you compete against yourself, you always win. You can't lose when you compete against yourself.

Learn instinctive, confidence-building tricks. Timely changes in goals when in a rut can work wonders. Sometimes, adding weight when in a rut helps because you have a built-in excuse and no pressure. You know it's your best weight ever, so past failures are erased from your mind. In 1975 I was stuck for months at a maximum bench press of 295 pounds. Three hundred was a major psych job for me. I finally increased the weight to 305 and had no pressure or past failures in my mind. The weight flew up with no problem the first time I tried it.

It's also very helpful to get angry. You must attack the weights as if they were going to attack your family. You're going to war with the weights. It's not, however, only a matter of positive thinking—you must combine anger with the positive thinking. If you saw the movie "The Water Boy," it gave some extreme and even hilarious examples of channeling anger in a positive way and illustrates what I mean.

Channel your frustrations into the exercise. Not only will you be stronger, you'll reduce your stress level and be more relaxed later. Channel anger or frustration towards the exercise, not towards yourself. Give it your best effort and then move to the next exercise. Don't sulk or whine if you didn't hit the goal. Just do your best and then drop it; otherwise your next set will be affected. Remember that Babe Ruth struck out 1,330 times and hit 714 home runs. The strange thing is that no one remembers the strikeouts. The thing to remember is that The Babe kept swinging the bat. If you keep giving honest effort, you'll get your dues in terms of poundage increases.

Think of yourself as big and strong, even if you're not yet. Use power thinking, not weak thinking. You are what you think about and will be dictated by your most dominant thoughts. Don't think of yourself as being genetically disadvantages, etc. Don't limit yourself. Have realistically high expectations. Aim high.

Have goals. You can't hit a target if you don't have one. Write down your goals and dwell on them. I repeat—write them down. One of the biggest traits of underachievers is that they never put their goals on paper. Believe you'll achieve your goals and most likely you will. Remember Henry Ford's quote: "Whether you think you can or think you can't, you're right!" That sums it up well. Much has been written about the power of belief. Any mental techniques without true belief are worthless.

Visualize good hard workouts. Complete many workouts in your head. Never miss lifts in your mind. Find time each day to go over a planned workout in your head. Dream creatively and see yourself breaking new personal records—feel them, see them, and smell them. See yourself as a winner, respected, and a champion. Know the difference between confidence and arrogance. Being confident and feeling good about yourself are great, but treat others with respect. Don't look up or down at anyone but straight in the eye.

The most important language you have is the one you use to talk to yourself. What you say to yourself and what you believe about yourself can have miraculous as well as devastating effects. What you say, think, and believe about yourself affects not only your cognitive thinking but also your subconscious mind. Your subconscious mind is extremely powerful and is essentially your emotional personality.

Never use negative language to yourself. When Tony Gwynn strikes out, he doesn't say "I suck" or "I can't hit." He says, "I wasn't at my best today but expect to be ready tomorrow." This is a good example of positive self-talk. Your subconscious mind is much larger than your conscious thinking mind. You can't say negative things about yourself without getting hurt.

BOB WHELAN'S Q&A

July 2002

Q. *How does an elliptical exerciser compare with a stairclimber and a treadmill? Which do you prefer, and why?*

A. I'm going to answer this question assuming that you're involved in some form of strength training. That being the case, cardiovascular exercise is only measured by two things: heart rate and time. As long as you can maintain the same heart rate for the same amount of time, then it really doesn't matter what specific type of cardio exercise you do. The type only matters if you're *not* strength training with weights. Then you would have to consider the muscular benefits of the cardio exercise.

Thirty years ago, back when few people lifted weights, many of the slogans we still hear now were born. Slogans like "swimming is the best exercise" and "walking is the best exercise." There's no "best" exercise. To be totally fit, you must strength train, stretch, *and* do cardiovascular exercise. Since most people didn't lift weights back then, they would consider an exercise like swimming to be the best exercise because your upper body would get some work too, unlike from jogging. Walking was only considered "the best" because more people could do it (but this was really nothing more than society having low standards).

Many people who should know better give all the wrong reasons for choosing a specific cardio exercise. It's a major mistake to rate a cardio exercise based on the very limited muscular benefits it gives. The muscular benefits from cardio exercise are so limited that I actually don't even consider them. You already have the muscular exercise benefits taken care of from your strength training, so the cardio exercise should only be rated for the benefits of fat burning and working the most important muscle of all, the heart. Find cardio exercise that you like and that doesn't injure or

267

bother you.

I personally like the stairclimber. I feel comfortable with it and like to compete with the machine. Is it the best? No, only the best for me because I'll do it. It works my heart and burns fat, which are the only reasons I do cardio (since I lift weights).

Once again, the best cardio exercise for you is the one that you will do.

Q. *I've been trying to get to the big 300 on my bench press for years, and I'm stuck at 250. what tips could you give to get me closer to my goal of a 300-pound bench press?*

A. Of course you should follow the general training guidelines such as getting enough recovery, lifting hard and heavy, eating well, and not overtraining. The advice I'm going to give you is beyond that and more like specific fine tuning.

When I was powerlifting, I was a double-bodyweight bencher— 365 at 181. this was done drug-free and without a bench shirt. I also coached powerlifting and learned that a lot of little things can make a big difference in your numbers. There are some techniques that most good benchers take for granted but less experienced lifters don't even notice. Sometimes the common training literature doesn't help because it's usually written for the beginner and doesn't fully explain certain details. It commonly just gives general information to steer you in the right direction. The general information, although helpful to many people, frequently ignores small details that can make a world of difference to lifters beyond the beginner stage. Here are a few tips that have helped me and my lifters:

1. Gripping the Bar

Hold the bar low on your palms near your wrist, not your fingers. This is the reason why some people swear by the thumbless grip because this grip ensures that the bar will stay low on your palms with the weight more in a direct line down your forearms. I'm not saying that you should use a thumbless grip (where the thumbs rest alongside the index fingers rather than around the bar and overlapping the tips of some of the fingers). I've never liked the thumbless grip, don't advocate it, and consider it dangerous. The reason for it being used is why I'm pointing this out. I always use a grip with my thumb around the bar and over the tips of one or two of my fingers, but you have to experiment with how you grip the bar so that it doesn't fall in your palm near your fingers.

Many people grip the bar too tightly and force it into an unfavorable position. You don't want the bar to bend your hand backwards too much. Ideally, you want your hands closer to straight up, not bent back. You want the weight to be transferred directly down your forearm. You may have to loosen your grip a little or slightly change the gripping angle of your hands to accomplish this, but it's very important if you're to have a good bench press.

2. Breathing

Even though we've all heard that you shouldn't hold your breath while lifting and to exhale on exertion, the way that you exhale can have a major impact on your lifting strength. It's not as simple as just inhaling on the negative part of the lift (eccentric) and exhaling on the positive side of the lift (concentric). Good lifters usually instinctively know that they need to have a slight delay exhaling (until the concentric part of the lift is almost complete).

You actually do hold your breath for a split second at the beginning of the concentric phase of the lift, only exhaling at the top of the concentric phase. This allows the diaphragm to remain rigid and tensed and provides a solid platform for the muscles to push from while lifting the weight.

If you simply start exhaling at the very bottom of the lift, the moving diaphragm provides no foundation to push from and you'll not lift as much weight.

This is advanced information. I'm not advocating that you hold your breath while lifting—just have a slight delay in exhaling—so listen carefully. You inhale coming down, hold your breath as the bar touches your chest, and hold your breath very briefly until the bar is near the completion of the lift; exhale as you complete the concentric part of the lift. There's just a slight delay in the exhaling part, that's ll.

3. Flex/Pop Your Lats

Many people don't realize that the lats can have a major impact on the bench press. You should pop or explode your lat muscles into action as you drive up the weight. Your lat explosion will move your shoulders forward and can have a major impact on getting the bar moving off your chest.

4. Thinking

Remember that during the actual repetition, you're not thinking about how your muscles "feel" when trying to lift heavily. You're thinking *functional* and only about getting the weight lifted. It's an entirely different way of thinking than when you're lifting using an intentional slow speed. Especially on low reps or singles, you should be thinking to explode the bar off your chest when benching.

We're talking about heavy weights here, so even "exploding" the weight will not actually come up fast. The heavy poundage will take care of that. So-called "explosive lifting" that's described as dangerous by some is different from what I'm referring to. The dangerous explosive lifting is usually done with a weight that's too light to explode with. You should only be thinking to explode with very heavy weights done for low reps or singles.

5. Become Robotic in Your Benching Style

Practice touching the same spot on your chest every time. Many people bench press by lowering the bar too high on their chests. To bench press heavily, have the bar touch at the nipples or below every time. Once you find your groove, use the same technique every time, pause, and drive up. Become almost robotic in your bench pressing style, creating a power groove. Motor learning and neurological pathways will become advanced as you find your strength groove. You'll also have less chance of getting injured when you do it exactly the same way every time, paying attention to important minor details.

Never bounce the bar off your chest, and don't even do "touch and go" benches. If you compete, you should practice bench pressing stricter than the strictest judge you've ever had or are ever likely to have. This means a pause at the chest for longer than one full second. Practice like this and then you'll have no fear. No matter how long they make you pause at the meet, it doesn't matter because you train every bench workout even stricter.

That's the way I did it. I didn't care who the judge was. Whenever I heard the judge clap in a meet, I thought I hadn't paused long enough compared to my usual training style. I almost felt like I cheated because my training was so much stricter. You should bench press with a distinct pause at the chest 'til the bar is motionless, then flex the lat muscles and drive up the weight as fast as possible.

6. Lower the Bar Slowly

Many inexperienced lifters try to get the lift over with as fast as possible, thinking that momentum and bouncing the bar off their chests will help. If you lower the bar too fast, then besides damaging your ribs, you'll also create a whiplash effect that actually makes the weight heavier. When you push up suddenly after coming down too fast, the bar is still going downward at the ends near the plates (and actually bends) while the center near the hands are trying to go up. Good benchers know that the bar will actually feel lighter if they lower it slowly.

Q. *I've seen arguments concerning the use of partial movements in a power rack, both for and against. Do you recommend/advocate any specific exercises for partials? Can partials really hold benefit in comparison to their full-range counterparts? And what personal experience do you have of partials?*

A. Like so many other questions, this one depends on the goals of the lifter, age, health, medical condition, history of injuries, etc. Would I recommend partials for a middle-aged businessman who wants to increase his strength mainly for health benefits? No, there's no reason to do so, and I wouldn't want to take the risk or responsibility for doing it. But if a guy seriously wants to compete as a strength athlete or even a regular guy who just loves training and is a seasoned lifter, healthy, committed, and serious about lifting as heavily as possible, then I would advocate some use of partials.

I've said before that I think partials can be helpful for certain people (e.g., seasoned lifters who want to do them and can do them with minimum risk) *when done in conjunction with or as an addition to the regular full range of-motion work.* I don't believe in partials as a replacement for full-range work but as a supplement for work on sticking points.

I've worked with partials on the bench press. After all the regular sets were done, I would do several partial sets with the pins set in the area of the sticking pt. I found them to be very helpful.

Q. *How's your training going, Bob?*

A. I've just recently gone back to the roots of my first 32 years of lifting. I'm now doing exclusively heavy low-rep barbell training after about five years of mostly machine training in which I spent almost two years training using slow speeds and doing just one set to failure. I really missed the clanging of the big plates, and my training now feels energized. It's an adjustment to say the least.

Motor learning is specific, that's for sure. My first few workouts were very light and I was very sore. The weights felt heavy, as I'd not lifted like this for a long time. Is it better? No. I just needed a change. I'm sure I'll use the machines again in the future, but for now I'm enjoying something else. That's what training is all about. You should enjoy it and not be afraid to try different things. I'm glad I trained on slow reps for two years and used mostly machines for five years. Now I can write about it and know what I'm talking about, unlike some who say the slow stuff is for wimps when they have no clue.

After about six weeks of going back to strictly barbell work using mostly low reps, I'm still lagging a little behind in upper-body strength but I'm about 90% back. I switched to doing front squats several months earlier and am getting some pretty good numbers. I trained for a goal of 300 for 20 reps in the front squat and came close but kept dumping the bar at about 16 reps with 300. I couldn't keep it on my shoulders long enough. I've switched to lower reps and want to see how close I can get to 400 for 5 reps. That's my goal, for now at least.

Q. *You've said that you like thick bars mainly for pulling movements. Do they have any real benefit for pushing movements? Also, how can you lift heavily with the thick bars without your grip giving out before your targeted upper-body muscle?*

A. Thick bars are a good tool to use to supplement your training so long as you don't get carried away with them. Most lifting bars have had thinner diameters for about 90 years now, for good reason. Most muscles are more effectively targeted with thinner handles because you can lift heavier weights without your grip

273

giving out first.

There are only limited exercises where you can really use thick bars productively, such as variations of curls, slow speed pulling movements (with lighter weights), and the second part of super-setted movements (with the heavier set done first with a thin-handled bar).

I have custom-made thick handles (that slide over the regular handle) for a lot of my pulling machines. For example, we'll go to failure on the Hammer Iso Row with the thick handles. When they hit "grip failure" (usually before failure of the other involved musculature), I pop off the thick handles. The clients give their hands a quick shake and then keep going until failure of the targeted muscles using the standard handles.

Thick handles are good, but you must use them wisely. You don't want to use them in a way that they give inferior work to the targeted muscles in the name of grip work.

For pushing movements, two-inch thick bars/handles don't really do much at all for the grip, but for many people they are actually more comfortable to use than the thinner-handled bars. The thicker handle forces the weight to be distributed deeper down on your palms near the wrist. It's ironic that most thick-handled bars don't make the pushing movement harder but actually more comfortable and easier.

Q. *When is the best time to do cardiovascular exercise? Is it better to do it on days when not strength training, or is it better before or after strength training on the same day?*

A. The main thing is that you get it done. If you do no cardiovascular exercise, that's much worse than any shortcomings I point out in any answers I could give to these questions, so keep that in mind.

The answers will depend a lot on your schedule and what you're able to do. Ideally, if you're able, it would be better to do cardio on different days from your weights. If you're doing strength training about twice per week, then you should try to make that your priority on those days. You have five other days to get the cardio work done. That's what I prefer. Strength training is enough to get done in a busy day.

But nothing is perfect and our schedules sometimes don't allow us to plan like we want. If you have to do your cardio on the same day as your weights work, that's okay. It's better than missing the cardio. Try to do it after your strength training. If you do it before, then your strength training will probably suffer. You'll probably have less energy and feel weaker, so I'd try to do the strength training first. But remember, getting it done any way is better than missing it completely.

BOB WHELAN'S Q&A

September 2002

Q. *I need some advice on the front squat. Is it a good alternative to the regular (back) squat? What's the best grip to use?*

A. In my opinion, the front squat is a *great* exercise. It's one of the most underrated of the good exercises. Most people. Just do the regular back squat and don't even consider the front squat. The front squat is still a squat, and it really makes no difference if you do it or the back squat version as far as your routine goes. It's more a matter of tradition that most people do back squats, though front squats are more tricky to perform than regular squats. It's my opinion that the front squat is at least as good or better—unless, of course, you're competing as a powerlifter, but even then it will take a minimum adjustment to switch over to the regular squat with no loss of strength; I've done it. Do what you like and prefer. If you prefer regular back squats, do them. They can be great, too.

Many feel, me included, that the front squat is an even harder version of the squat than the regular one. I've done the front squat for years, with back squats, too. I only do front squats now because back squats hurt my neck area. Every time I back squat, I end up with a stiff neck and can't turn my head for a few days. I think I'm getting a warning following decades of heavy weights on my spine. Everyone is different, so if you like front squats, just replace the back squats with them. No big deal. You're doing no less work, that's for sure, and maybe even more work.

Ask Olympic lifters about front squats. You use less weight as you must stand straight or else you'll dump the bar. It makes you use better form and is more leg specific and less back-and-glute specific than the back squat.

You don't actually grip the bar during the front squat. My

fingertips just touch the bar and keep it in place. The bar rests in a groove in my delts, and my fingers must help keep it there. There's no gripping involved. If you're in a power rack—which you should be for the front squat, with pins set in place to catch the bar if you have to dump it—you've nothing to worry about. Just get your balance and form down pat first, and then build up the weight.

Many non-Olympic lifters like the cross-arms method. Olympic lifters usually don't use cross-arms when front squatting, since cross-arms are not used in Olympic lifting. I don't cross my arms. Use what feels comfortable to you. Remember, the bar is supported in a groove in your deltoids. Once you find what feels comfortable and you can keep good form and balance, then you should be able to up the poundage quickly. Again, take your time to master form with a light weight before you go increasing the poundage.

The style that you use to support the bar (cross-armed or Olympic) is really not that important, as it's not actually involved in lifting the weight. I sometimes do a technique demo for my clients. I do a little job with a light bar on my shoulders to show how the bar is wedged in my delts. I then do some front squats with my arms out straight just to demonstrate that the key is bar positioning and balance and has nothing to do with grip. On the final few reps, due to total body fatigue, you must resist slouching on your form. You'll need to strain to hold good form in order to get the last few reps. Gravity pulls you forward with the weight, and it's harder to stay straight up when you're tired. This is when your fingertips might help hold the bar in place. Sometimes I try "one too many" and end up dumping the bar in the rack.

Some people, especially those new to the front squat, may feel more comfortable with a secure grip on the bar while squatting. Check out AtomicAthletic.com, as they now have a seven-foot bar weighing 52 pounds that has parallel-grip handles made especially for front squatting. Ken Mannie, strength coach at Michigan State University, has his charges front squat with this bar, and he loves the feel of the bar while front squatting. A bar with this grip may solve your gripping problem while front squatting.

Q. *The upright row is considered a dangerous exercise by some. What's your opinion of this exercise?*

A. As I've gotten older, I've developed an appreciation of Stuart McRoberts' conservative approach to form and exercise selection. I used to do the upright row with my hands close together and pull the bar all the way up to my chin. It never bothered me when I was younger, but it does now. I still do it (but differently) and think it's a good exercise as long as you don't pull the bar up too high and don't use a close grip. I believe it becomes increasingly dangerous if you go above the lower chest level.

I always do a few warm-up sets in the upright row before the heavy sets. For both warm-up and work sets, I keep my hands right on the edge of the knurl mark on a York bar (about 16 inches apart). I lower the bar slowly with a good bottom pause and raise it no higher than chest/nipple level. If you do the movement this way, your chances of injury are dramatically reduced. Of course, if you still get a negative reaction even to the modified version, eliminate the exercise. Never persist with any exercise that causes pain or any other type of negative reaction.

Q. *Some people recommend training the grip hard once or at most twice a week, but a few recommend training it almost every day, rotating a number of different exercises. How much is enough with grip work, and should the grip be worked more frequently than other bodyparts?*

A. I may be the wrong person to ask this question of, as I do grip work just to assist my strength training, not to compete in any form of grip competition. It may be different if you're seriously training to excel in a grip competition or demonstration, such as closing a certain gripper. I recommend doing your grip training just like you would any other muscle—hitting it twice every 7-10 days per the "commandments" of WST. Why should the grip get any special extra attention, unless you're really involved in grip competition, which I'm not and neither are my clients.

It's great if you have a strong grip, but your major lifts should be as impressive, if not more so. I get a good chuckle when I see some of the guys who are so into grip work that they seem to forget they have a body attached to their hands. I know a guy who can almost close the number three gripper, which is very impressive and a lot better than I can do, but he can bench press only about 250 pounds and squat maybe 350 if he's lucky. He thinks he's a strong guy just because of his grip.

I think some people are getting their priorities mixed up. Work your whole body, which includes the grip. Don't put emphasis on the grip at the expense of the major strength-training movements. People who can only do feats of strength with the grip aren't real strongmen, in my opinion. If their squat, bench press, deadlift, military press, etc., are done with heavy weights *and* they have a strong grip, to me, that's impressive. To have a really strong grip and be weak in the major barbell movements is getting it all wrong.

Q. *What do you think of the book* Muscletown USA *by John D. Fair?*

A. In my opinion, although it unfairly treats Hoffman too negatively, Fair's book is excellent. It's full of historical information and is a fascinating read. The facts in it can't be disputed, but some of the negative things about Hoffman were unfairly portrayed. The same effort wasn't made to dig in detail into the personal lives of other major characters in Iron Game history. I don't know of any new book coming out with a more positive spin on the York/Hoffman side, but I'd love to see it.

The problem is that Fair seems to go out of his way to show Hoffman's bad side. He seemed biased towards Joe Weider and cynical/negative about Hoffman. Factual information can still be unfair. People usually dig deeper into personal negative things if they don't like you and omit some of the positive things. (The opposite applies if they like you.) if you can keep that in mind, *Muscletown USA* is a great book.

I love Hoffman. His influence got me started in all this when I bought my first copies of *Muscular Development* and *Strength and Health* in 1964 when I was ten years old. I admire the man and won't let Fair's book change my admiration for Hoffman.

Q. *What's the best description of how the old-timers really trained?*

A. The only real absolute about the old-timers is that they trained naturally, hard, and progressively. They may have had crude equipment and limited information, but they made the most of what they had. If you take a close look at old Iron Game literature, you'll find a common theme: health, strength, vigor, and longevity. Cosmetic results, although mentioned, were clearly secondary. The cosmetic results were believed to be the end result of "doing the right thing" and were a reward for effort, discipline, and a lifestyle commitment.

The titles of the popular books and magazines reflected these values. There were *Strength and Health, Health and Strength, Physical Culture, Strength, The Strong Man,* and numerous other titles. Compare these titles to the best-selling training books and magazines of today—the difference is astounding.

The pioneers of Physical Culture were not just body beautiful posers. They were strong! Eugene Sandow and others competed in various feats of strength. They had to make do with crude training facilities and equipment, but they made the most of what they had. They had to endure the wrath of society, as attaining health and strength was not a trendy thing to do in those days. This is how the term *health nut* got started (they were definitely not called buff!). even though they had far less information available, they swore by the information they did have.

How many of us truly can say we're using the information we have? Jack LaLanne was so dedicated that he trained his mind to visualize disgusting images at the very thought of junk food. Cosmetic results were seen as the reward for correct living and hard training.

Many of our Physical Culture forefathers went beyond physical health and were concerned with mental and spiritual health as well. Peary Rader frequently wrote articles about spiritual health; Bob Hoffman and Bernarr MacFadden, in addition to writing about training, wrote about practically everything dealing with health and happiness, including moral issues.

We now have much better overall equipment, gyms, and nutritional and health knowledge. But we also have the horrendous mess of drug abuse. Public acceptance of and involvement in training is much higher now. But most of the training principles have been around a long time.

There's nothing really new as far as strength-training principles are concerned. It just gets repackaged. Read the "Letters from Chas" on NaturalStrength.com and his articles in old issues of *Hardgainer* as he repeatedly covers this topic. There's no single training philosophy that defines the old-timers. Klein, Maxick, Cyr, and Grimek trained differently, just as individuals today train differently. Chas stated that none of today's training principles are really new. The only exception I can think of that may be considered new is the concept of *very* slow speed training.

Q. *I'm curious as to what you think about Arthur Jones, his writing, and strength training methods. Also, do you consider yourself an advocate of HIT?*

A. I have a great deal of respect for Jones and consider him to be one of the brightest minds in the history of strength training. I didn't discover him right away, though. My early influences were mainly from York (Hoffman and Grimek), Brad Steiner, and later from the original *Iron Man* from Peary Rader. In the late 1970s, I was temporarily influenced a great deal by *Heavy Duty* from Mike Mentzer but later realized that he just paraphrased and repackaged Arthur Jones' theories, so it was really Jones I was influenced by. I don't agree with everything Jones says but most of it. He definitely had a big impact on my beliefs.

I frequently use multiple sets, low reps, and barbells. I believe how you train depends on the goal of your training. A powerlifter has to do low reps, multiple sets, and use a barbell. A basketball player doesn't. I don't believe you have to go to failure to get good results so long as you train progressively. It depends on the goal of your training and your circumstances.

When it comes to training stimulus, I'm mainly a poundage guy. A lot of HIT guys never talk about poundage; it's always only about going to failure. I always put poundage (in good form) first, ahead of going to failure or anything else as far as training stimulus goes. Although I'm a big supporter of going to failure and controlled speed of motion training (for some trainees), for me they are clearly secondary to load progression.

I have a broad view of strength training and can see many ways that work. I don't feel the need to try to persuade people to do exactly what I do, nor do I get personally offended by differences in training philosophy other than those that use drug support. The most important thing is that you're natural and trying to train hard and lift heavier. If so, we're brothers, and there's no need to argue about minor details.

In strength training, it's all good as long as you follow sensible rules of safety, progression, and recovery. If you do power cleans or don't do them, I don't care so long as you don't get hurt. Same with odd objects, going to failure, etc. just don't get injured!

I see the various modes and methods of strength training as tools in a tool chest. A craftsman can collect and use many tools to perform his art. Only a fool would throw useful tools away and insist on using just a few tools. Different tools can be used for different people. Some need low reps and multiple sets due to their goals, and some need one set to failure.

Regardless of the method used in strength training, I always put the greatest emphasis on load or poundage progression. Effort without progression is no better than calisthenics or manual labor.

BOB WHELAN'S Q&A

November 2002

Q. *Have you seen lifters who've g*otten a lot stronger but not much *more "muscular"? And what about the reverse where a trainee looks muscular but isn't strong? If so, how do you account for* this?

A. The vast majority of the time, muscular size and strength go hand in hand. Usually when you see a guy who looks real strong, he is! I would say this would be the case for the vast majority of readers, because they are natural and train properly with the basic exercises.

Looking very strong doesn't always mean being muscular as defined by mainstream society. It should mean hardened and balanced thickness in the right areas. Usually, when you train for strength, muscular development and size come with it. I'm talking about balanced muscular size, not the phony biceps-and-chest-only size to impress the saloon patrons.

I've seen cases where trainees look muscular by mainstream standards but aren't nearly as strong as people would think. They usually don't train for strength. They don't have the balanced *look of power* from heavy, hard training with the basic exercises. They look like what Dr. Ken calls "a collection of bodyparts." They don't have the thickness in the back, hips, neck, traps and legs. Leg development is the sign of a true serious lifter. If a guy's legs are underdeveloped (and he has no legitimate knee or back problem), he's simply not going to be strong. He's not serious and hasn't paid his dues. He doesn't know the meaning of hard training.

Some of those who look muscular as defined by most of society are surprisingly weak when put to the test of strength. This is because they usually train on isolation exercises and yet can still get artificially big due to steroid use.

The words *strength* and *muscular* are loosely used these days. They usually have more to do with low bodyfat than anything functional. Some of the worst offenders are the media and the so-called "fitness pros." It's their influence that's unfortunately getting many well-intentioned beginners off to a bad start.

The politically correct climate of today tends to de-emphasize anything masculine. Since strength and manhood have a close historical connection, the definition of the terms *strength* and *muscle* have been cleverly repackaged. People have been brainwashed to associate being defined, cut, ripped (or simply having a low bodyfat percentage) with being strong and muscular. With this new definition, all sorts of gimmicks can now be targeted at men and women of all ages.

The term *strength*, properly used, could describe a 500-pound squat. Being strong doesn't mean looking like the latest Hollywood stud on a nightly tabloid show. The terms *strong* and *muscular* today are indeed commonly used to define only a certain cut or ripped look. Movie stars are called muscular when they are nothing but good abs, low bodyfat and a tan.

Strength is correctly defined as "the ability to produce force." When you acquire this ability you build strong, thick muscles that can't be missed. You also build thickness of ligaments, tendons and bones—your tan and bodyfat percentage are irrelevant. No matter what you wear or at what angle you're seen, you look strong—it's unmistakable! You look as powerful in a raincoat as in a tank top. You look as massive from behind as you do from the front. A properly trained individual is thick from a side view.

Heavy pushing and pulling consistently done over the years adds inches to the front and back of the torso, hips and legs. It's impossible for well-trained individuals to hide the fact that they look strong. Because of this confidence, they walk around relaxed and graceful, unlike the insecure underdeveloped (but cut) guys who try to look flexed at all times. The latter individuals give us a bad name. they give the impression to the general public that it's because they train with weights that they are so stiff and awkward.

You can spot a mile away those who avoid the basic multi-joint exercises. These individuals train almost exclusively on isolation exercises and show it by their uneven muscular development. They usually don't work their legs much, and only like to train their arms or chest. Their muscles don't blend or seem to belong together. They usually have one good bodypart that stands out and appears to have been surgically transplanted to a normal body. They are dumfounded when you ask them about progression. They don't have a clue as to the meaning of strength.

In my view, true serious lifters love to train hard and hear the clanging and rattling of heavy iron when big plates are loaded. The harder the exercise, the more they like it. They focus on the basic movements because they know that they work. When you do the basic movements, your muscles work and grow together. You're naturally more symmetrical because you're training your whole body hard.

If you take a look at the rugged builds of the old timers, you'll notice that they had symmetry. They trained all the major muscle groups hard and heavy with a wide variety of multi-joint exercises, many of which are not commonly done today. Look at the thickness of the traps, glutes, legs, back and forearms of George Jowett! You don't get this from doing only isolation exercises. No matter what Jowett wore, he looked huge and powerful. When muscle and strength are correctly built, you can't hide it. While

Jowett had great genetics for strength, his training was essential for developing his muscle and strength.

If you read some of the old muscle classics, you'll frequently find mention of the word *sinews*. We now call them tendons. To build tendon strength, you must lift heavy and pay your dues. Tendons only get thicker from heavy poundages.

There are some rare cases where you'll find someone who correctly trains for strength and gets stronger but doesn't seem to grow much in size. If this is a beginner we're talking about, the explanation may be a genetic one. For advanced trainees, there are several other factors to consider.

Trainees who compete in a weight class and have to abide by weight restrictions make a conscious effort to get stronger and stay in a given weight class. They usually do very low reps and singles which some research indicates have a lower corresponding ratio to hypertrophy than moderate-range reps do. The second factor could be an improvement in motor unit function or the neurological adaptations to training. The third would be an improvement in the mental aspects of training and/or motivation. The fourth factor would be artificial performance enhancement—i.e., better assistance gear, drugs, etc. The fifth factor would be an improvement in technique or skill.

Q. *What do you think of dipping and chinning for increased reps, with no additional weight, for muscle growth, as an alternative to low-to-medium reps and increasing poundage?*

A. Chins and dips are hard enough so that many if not most people, especially beginners, will not have to add weights. The reps with bodyweight alone are probably not going to be high.

Chins and dips are two of the best exercises you can do for the development of the upper body. Dips are a major pushing movement, and chins are a major pulling movement, so this combination of exercises alone will work the major muscle groups of the upper body.

If you're getting high reps on these exercises in good form, it would be better to add additional weight if you're strength training and not just focusing on general fitness, conditioning, or muscular endurance. You'll still build muscle with high-rep sets with only bodyweight, but the corresponding ratio of muscle size and strength is higher if you train progressively by increasing the load.

Many types of training will build some strength and muscular development, but they are inferior to load-progression strength training. Bodyweight exercises alone will get you stronger for sure and will build muscle. For many this is the best form of training. For example, if you're a wrestler and constantly use bodyweight leverages as the primary test of strength, the use of bodyweight exercises may be optimal. You're using a different type of strength in your sport. Your strength isn't going to be tested like it is for a powerlifter. Wrestling, although requiring strength, isn't as strength focused as powerlifting, Olympic lifting, or strongman competitions where progressive strength training would be far more beneficial.

High bodyweight reps with no progression (or additional load added to bodyweight) will build muscle and strength for sure, but will mainly build muscular endurance which, for some, is perfect. Remember that strength is the ability to produce force. Muscular endurance is how many times you can do something at a sub-maximal rate of force.

It all depends on your goal for training. If you truly want to get as strong and muscular as possible, then load-progressive strength training is far more beneficial than bodyweight exercises along where there's no weight progression.

Q. *How do you train to become more focused on the moment at hand, say during the execution of a lift? I sometimes stray mentally for a brief second, and that's enough to undermine the effort. The mental aspect of lifting seems to be one of my largest pitfalls.*

A. To recap what I've recommended before, here are some tips. This is an important topic, hence, why it's being covered again.

1. Think of a time limit target for going all-out. If you're going for a maximum single, tell yourself that you're going to go all-out and, for just a few seconds, nothing else exists but this exercise. "I'll explode like a bomb for a few seconds, and then come back to sanity." For just a few seconds you'll channel *everything* into this. If it's a set, substitute "All I have to do is go all-out for less than a minute." A time ceiling helps your mind target the intensity better, at least for me.

2. Take about 20 seconds before you lift and think about what you're doing—no talking for at least 20 seconds.

3. Take the pressure off by telling yourself that this is fun and the worst thing that can happen is you just miss the lift—nothing else. There's really *no pressure*. It's fun. Attack the weights with focused and controlled aggression like you've got nothing to lose. Sometimes people worry so much about *not getting a lift*. This ruins concentration. Again, don't worry about not getting it, it's just fun. Think about getting it and well on *that*.

4. Read the articles I've written for the "Mind Strength" section on my website, www.naturalstrength.com.

Q. *How would you modify a strength-training program to accommodate someone who works at a very demanding physical job—eight hours a day pulling and pushing on heavy industrial tools?*

A. You can still train hard, so I'm not going to hand out excuses. Many of us work hard, so a lot of this could be in your head. Working hard on the job is a good thing and what you're supposed to do. Here's some simple advice for you: I would cut back your training to two whole-body workouts in a ten-day period and only do *one hard work set* after warm-ups, per exercise.

Q. *My lateral delts are lagging behind the rest of my shoulders. I do variations of the press. How can I bring my lateral delts up to par?*

A. Add lateral raises with dumbbells to your routine. This should round out your shoulders. I've never said *not* to do isolation exercises. As long as you do the core compound movements, you can add a few isolation exercises to your routine if you feel you need them and are able. What I'm against is *replacing* the basic compound movements with isolation exercises. The *core foundation* of your routine remains the basic, multi-joint movements.

Q. *Is it possible to get good results if you train the whole body three times a week, but on a heavy-light-medium format? Isn't this how many people used to train in the pre-steroids era?*

A. This depends on how you design your program, what your goals are, and what you enjoy. Of course, it's possible that some people may train three times per week in a heavy, light and medium format with great results. You can also train three times per week with very abbreviated workouts, without any heavy-light-medium format. Most of the guys I know and respect who train the whole body three times per week have a much shorter and less intensive workout than the kind we do at WST. That's why they can do it three times per week. It's designed for three times per week. The WST type workout is designed for twice every 7-10 days. Neither is better. They both work but are designed to work on a different schedule. With the heavy-light-medium way, you're actually training heavy only once per week, so is it really more work? It depends on how you look at it. Try the different methods and use which works best for you and that you enjoy. Both can work well as long as you eat right, get plenty of rest, and train progressively.

The type of training we do at WST wouldn't work on a three-times-per-week schedule. That's because we go heavy and hard every time, with moderate volume, so you need more time to recover. We usually do multiple sets, most of them to failure (and sometimes beyond, with forced reps), with as heavy a weight as possible that good form allows. We work the whole body including neck, grip, and abs. the workout is about one hour, with most of the time spent working, not resting. We take very little rest. In fact, more than two minutes is considered luxurious. I will sometimes say to my (non-beginner) clients, "Take a long luxurious three-minute rest."

I design exercise sequences so the prime movers get plenty of rest between hits, for maximum performance even with little overall rest. We usually do a three-in-a-row no-rest sequence like push-pull-legs, then rest for 2-3 minutes, then do either neck, abs or grip, and repeat the sequence. This gives a few minutes after the leg movement—where rest is most needed—but gives the muscles more built-in rest from the sequence's design while still keeping the overall intensity high and getting a lot of work done in an hour. You're drenched in sweat at the end of the workout and dead tired. You need three or four days to recover.

It's not a matter of *choosing* not to do this routine three times per week. You just *can't* do it three times per week. It's not designed for three times per week. The toughest, most in-shape, hard-core guy is going to be physically unable to train with this WST type of workout more than twice in a 7-10 day period. You risk overtraining and perhaps injury if you do this workout like we do it but three or more times per week. You might be able to do it for a week to stubbornly/foolishly prove you could, but you wouldn't stick with it that way. Anyone who doesn't believe me is welcome to come to WST and let me train you on Monday; then I'll call you on Wednesday to see if you're ready to train again.

BOB WHELAN'S Q&A

January 2003

More About "Cuts"

Keeping your bodyfat low is healthy and important. The thing I don't like is confusing the purpose of strength training (and the definition of strength and being muscular) with other health issues. The purpose of strength training is to build muscle and strength. You don't lift weights for the purpose of producing definition or cuts. Stick to the same heavy and hard format with basic exercises to build muscle even if your goal is to be defined.

You have to have muscle in order to be muscular. If you look like a human anatomy chart or like you just got out of a concentration camp, you may have low bodyfat but you're not muscular. Lift weights to build muscle and strength but watch your diet and/or add cardiovascular training to reduce your bodyfat.

If you haven't built a lot of muscle over your whole body including your legs, glutes, traps, back and neck, you're not muscular. Being muscular doesn't mean simply having a low bodyfat like it's portrayed by many people today. Even a lot of "natural" bodybuilding contests are guilty of this misunderstanding. I recently saw some pictures of the winners at a "natural" bodybuilding contest, and they looked sickly thin and starved.

Q. *What precautions do you insist on if one of your clients has high blood pressure but his doctor's consent to exercise?*

A. The first thing I do is make sure that he really does have medical clearance to train. I try to find out if the doctor has any specific restrictions as far as exercise is concerned. If everything checks out and the trainee is free to train, I look at several health factors that may help lower blood pressure. I take a look at his bodyfat percentage, how much alcohol he drinks, stress factors in his life—e.g., job and family—ad how much cardiovascular exercise he's currently doing. (I won't train smokers since, to me, smoking is blasphemous to a training lifestyle and disrepectful to me as a coach.)

This answer can evolve into a lot of areas because high blood pressure could be related to many things. Everyone who's familiar with my writings knows that even though I advocate serious strength training, I've always recommended cardiovascular exercise and a "train for total health" concept, especially for non-competitive trainees over the age of 30, which happens to be the vast majority of individuals.

I usually recommend more cardio work than most strength writers who advocate only two cardiovascular workouts per week. I've always stood by the guidelines set by the American College of Sports Medicine, which is a minimum of three cardio workouts per week. For those who need to lose a lot of fat, I raise it to four or five times per week until the excess fat is lost. Then they can settle in on a three-times-per-week maintenance schedule.

For your cardiovascular exercise, anything that's safe is helpful, but the latest research shows that higher intensity or interval type cardio is far more beneficial than a longer but moderate intensity/comfortable workout. I now do shorter but more intensive cardio workouts. I used to use the Stairmaster for 45 minutes on a moderate setting. Now I do 30 minutes o the interval setting. Even though the workout is 15 minutes shorter, I'm working a lot harder and doing a lot of sprinting, with moderate recovery intervals in between. I just barely get my breath back and then it's time for another sprint. A half hour of this type of work is about all I can take. But you have to slowly work up to it and be careful. Don't kill yourself trying to get in shape too fast. Be patient and slowly up the intensity level.

Cardiovascular exercise is filled with a lot of confusing information. One confusing item that was even taught to me in school is that moderate intensity cardio workouts will burn more fat than intensive cardio work. This is really a play on words and not totally truthful.

You may burn more fat *directly* using moderate intensity work, as fat is the direct fuel used in this energy system. You'll burn more fat *indirectly* by burning more *overall* calories in the more intensive workout, *providing* you do it for long enough. Any calories burned, whether carbohydrates or fat, will eventually translate into more fat loss when an overall caloric debt is created. Your body balances the caloric debt by burning the stored bodyfat reserves, so in the long run you may burn more fat by the interval-type more intensive work.

Q. *How should a trainee alter training and eating habits as he/she ages?*

The older you get, the harder it is to keep fat off, at least for most people. You definitely have to adjust your diet and take cardiovascular exercise more seriously as you get older, especially when you see people your own age or even younger dropping dead from heart attacks.

Strength training along with cardiovascular exercise is optimal in order to lose fat. Strength training is far more important for fat reduction than previously thought by medical experts. Strength training builds muscle, which will increase fuel needs. Muscles are like the engine that moves your body. When you build a bigger engine, it needs more fuel. This is a good analogy to use to explain how your basal metabolic rate will be increased by strength training. You burn more calories even at rest because of the increased fuel/caloric needs of the larger muscles.

Strength training is also an enabler. Many people are unable to exercise when they get older. Strength training enables you to move around, be independent, and able to do cardio work. Strength training is also far more beneficial for your heart than previously thought. Strength training is now being rated just as important or even more important than cardio for your overall health. To be in optimal health, however, *do both.*

Many individuals, when young, had to "stuff their faces" at every sitting, drink a lot of milk, and eat cans of tuna and just about everything else in sight, every day, to gain muscular size. This was definitely the case for me. Some people mistakenly think I'm an easy gainer, or heavy boned, which is totally untrue. I weighed 115 pounds as a high school freshman and lifted and "stuffed my face" to get to about 155 as a senior at age 17.

I was naturally skinny and had to force myself to grow. I had to eat a lot at every meal and in between. I never had to worry about getting fat. I worried about being skinny. I had to eat like crazy just to maintain my bodyweight, and after a while it was ingrained in me to eat like a starved dog all the time. It became the normal way to eat for me. I would tell my friends that I was on a special "seafood diet." When they asked about it, I would tell them, "I see food and I eat it!"

In the US Air Force I had a friend, Ed Pimentel, who was a cook and had access to the food. Sometimes I would have two or three steaks and always had the best chow available because of my connections with Ed. The base usually only served steak once a week, but we could eat it in private after everyone left and the chow hall closed. But overall, the chow hall had good food every day, even without Ed. I had no problem with the military food and loved it. Back in the late seventies it was just sixty-five cents for breakfast, all you could eat; and one dollar and ten cents for each other meal, again all you could eat. I did get my money's worth, that's for sure. I build myself up to about 186 pounds from the great US Air Force food, and it was a solid 186. I would just reduce before a meet to get to the 181 class, which is where I usually lifted.

The point is this: When I got to my late thirties, around 37 or 38, I noticed a definite shift in my metabolism. I started putting on excess fat and had to start eating differently, or else I'd end up seriously obese. I can walk by a pizza now, just smell the pizza, and almost gain five pounds! Forget about me eating the pizza! Even if you can eat a lot without getting fat, still stick with healthy foods.

I spent the first 38 years of my life trying to gain or maintain my weight but have spent the last ten years either trying not to gain weight or to lose weight. As you get older, your body changes and you have to adjust to stay healthy. This goes for warming up, exercise selection, training volume and frequency, cardio and nutrition. I eat way less than I used to and do way more cardio and *still* have to watch my weight. *You definitely have to change your training and eating habits when you get older.*

I now do what I call extra triceps work by pushing the food away from me at the table. I usually only eat "like I used to" on special occasions like Thanksgiving, after the Clinic, or while visiting Drew Israel.

In addition to cardio training, I would also encourage individuals to see a registered dietician to get their diet in order, reduce alcohol consumption, and keep a positive attitude. A good multi-vitamin/mineral is also important. If you have high cholesterol, try to find a product with low iron or no iron, as latest research indicates a relationship between high iron and high cholesterol with heart attack in men. Also, the primary factors that raise HDL are exercise and niacin, so I'd be sure my multi-vitamin has a high niacin content.

Q. *I keep hearing about fiber types. What are your views about*

fiber typing and how it may affect training progress?

A. We're born with a certain number of short-term anaerobic fast twitch fibers (type IIb) and a certain number of aerobic slow twitch (type I) fibers. We also have an *intermediate* fiber type which is in the fast twitch (type II) group but geared more towards muscular endurance—type IIa fibers (*long-term* anaerobic). Some of these intermediate IIa fibers may be converted to type I or perhaps even type IIb fibers if the individual trains very hard in a specific way for a long period. For example, a marathon runner would probably have some of his type IIa fibers converted to type I fibers because of his extensive aerobic training. A powerlifter may have some of his intermediate fibers converted to type IIb fibers.

This helps to explain why it's impossible to be a world class powerlifter and a world class marathon runner at the same time. To be world class, you must have a very good heredity for the given activity. If you're to be a world class powerlifter, you would have to be born with a good percentage of fast twitch fibers in place to be developed. In addition to that, you would have a lot of genetically gifted competition, and you'd need to train extremely hard. This hard training may convert some of the intermediate fibers to type IIb fibers.

Some easy gainers with a higher fast twitch ratio are going to progress a lot faster than the hard gainer who has a higher slow twitch fiber ratio. But don't get discouraged. Being world class is one thing, but to improve greatly and be better than over 90% of society can be done by almost anyone who's healthy and willing to work. No matter what your genetics, you can be better than over 905 of society because the standards of society are so low.

Q. *Is the drug problem in competitive bodybuilding, powerlifting, Olympic lifting and strongman competitions getting better in recent years due to increased drug testing?*

A. No. if anything, the problem is getting worse. Don't be fooled by phony statistics. Drug use by athletes, especially Iron Game and strength athletes, is higher than ever. They are just not getting caught. There are now hundreds of drugs to improve performance. Many of them can't be detected because a test for them hasn't even been developed, e.g., human growth hormone, which is probably the most commonly used banned substance by elite athletes today. Even many of the drugs that can be tested for can be altered with masking agents so the athlete will usually still test clean.

The technology for beating drug tests and getting athletes to test clean is far ahead of the advances to catch the cheats. There are hundreds of crooked doctors, chemists, and self-trained (ex-bodybuilder type) steroid experts who get paid big bucks from bodybuilders, lifters, and all types of world class athletes to help them use drugs and get away with it. These drug gurus mix and develop custom "designer-type" steroids that are "stealth-like" and undetectable due to the masking agent that has altered the original drug.

There are even websites that are purely dedicated to help juicers avoid getting caught buying and using drugs.

Most steroid tests only work conclusively on pure, unaltered, commercially available steroids. The tester is looking for a very specific result for each drug tested. When the drug gurus mix these drugs, change them or alter them with masking agents, the results are clouded and inconclusive and fool the tester. Even the testers who are not fooled have to worry about lawsuits and proving a positive case if it goes to court.

Of course, it's not just steroids that are flagged in drug tests. In fact, it's often drugs other than steroids that get caught in tests. This isn't, however, because steroid use is on the way out but because the various authorities have to save face and look like they are doing something. The most important drug abuse isn't being tested for successfully.

Almost all testing is done with urine, not blood. Most experts agree that blood testing is more accurate than testing urine, and some of the drugs that are undetectable in urine can be found in blood. But blood has too many problems, as it clots and spoils, has to be kept cold, and to provide samples of it would be against the religious beliefs of many. Most people just don't want to handle blood because of contagious diseases, broken vials, etc. blood is a major headache to deal with. It's also a lot more expensive to test blood than urine. Then there are also the possible civil liberties lawsuits, as taking blood is considered a lot more invasive to someone's body.

Many governing bodies may also fear that if they switch to blood testing, the number of positive tests would rise sharply. This would hurt the public image of these governing bodies, not to mention their big bucks corporate sponsorships. The legal complications and fear of expensive lawsuits by the athletes have caused many drug tests to be merely a going-through-the-motions procedure. Many sports officials fear that some of the new drug testing methods may not stand up in a court of law.

Drug testing in general is also expensive, so low level competition can't afford it. Athletes could use drugs for several years before having to take a single test. By then, they can probably afford the more expensive stuff that can't be detected. Sadly, we can never again be sure that an athlete has prevailed by honest effort, sweat, and guts.

There are many people who are under the false impression that, due to the declining number of positive test results in the Olympics, NFL, and various Iron Game/strength sports, the drug problem is finally coming under control. Nothing could be further from the truth. The governing bodies and organizations of these sports would like you to believe the problem is coming under control. But they are more concerned with the image of the problem than the actual problem. The problem is worse than ever. Take a look at baseball. Every year, testing is becoming more and more of a joke, and now only the dumb athletes get caught.

BOB WHELAN'S Q&A

March 2003

Q. *When designing a program, what do you think is the right relationship between the bench press and the overhead press?*

A. I believe in treating them equally. They are in two different planes of motion, so do both for balanced strength. One is a vertical push (overhead press) and the other is a horizontal push (bench press). I see no reason (other than injury) to ignore one in favor of the other. It seems that many people have an extreme view of the bench press. They either love the exercise (and sometimes base their entire self-worth or strength self-esteem on it), or they totally ignore it in favor of the overhead press.

The latter rationalize that the overhead press builds more muscle or that the old-timers did the overhead press and most didn't do the supine bench press. Often, though, it's because they are just poor bench pressers and they can hide this weakness by just claiming "not to do the bench press."

I believe in a moderate but healthy view of the bench press. It shouldn't be the ego lift to size up one's strength, but neither should it be ignored. It's a good exercise. That's it—a good compound movement that should be done and not ignored.

A foolish reason for ignoring the bench press is that it's not a ground-based exercise. Just because your feet are on the ground doesn't make a lift better. Ground based lifts are not superior just because your feet are on the ground. Dirt, grass or floor does nothing for your strength. Many machines have metal platforms that you stand on. Is that ground based? Many upper-body exercises can't be ground based. Dips and chins aren't ground based since you're off the ground. Are they no good? Horizontal movements such as the bench press would be impossible to do

300

because of gravity if it wasn't for benches (or machines) to allow you to push from a horizontal position. The fact that your feet aren't on the floor (other than for stabilization purposes) has got nothing to do with it.

The bench press became popular in the mid-twentieth century. Prior to that, supine pressing on the floor was done but it wasn't popular or efficient due to the elbows only being able to go down to floor level. You can see pictures of a young John Grimek on the old Mark Berry wall charts doing the floor press with his elbows hitting the floor.

It may be hard to believe now, but using a bench wasn't common 'til about 50-60 years ago. Part of the reason for this was that training with weights wasn't popular then. They had fewer good gyms in the whole world than some big cities have today. Most people scoffed at lifting and had a negative opinion of it. Only a few companies made equipment for lifting and stuck mainly to barbells. Today, hundreds of companies make good equipment. Even mass production of adjustable barbells was new in the twentieth century.

Lifting weights was an obscure pastime done by so few people that the technological resources available weren't applied to it. (In addition, due to the World Wars, there were long periods when metal was scarce.)

Just because the old-timers didn't have benches available is no reason for *you* not to bench press. The old-timers had hardly any good gyms available and very little good equipment. Many of the old-timers had to use out-houses and had no indoor plumbing. Many of the old-timers smoked cigarettes because they didn't know any better. Do you want to go back to that also? The reason benches were eventually made is simple: *Progress!*

What's the reason that the bench press became so popular so fast? It went from nonexistent to king in just a few years. The reason is because it's a good exercise. It works and produces great results.

The simple use of the bench turned the hardly-ever-done floor press into one of the most popular exercises—the bench press.

Physical Culture isn't past tense. It's alive today and continues to improve and advance along with society. Imagine where we would be today if our Iron Game pioneers always looked to the past for answers. Be thankful that they were visionaries and applied the principles of Physical Culture to modern advances. The principles don't change, but the applications of those principles do.

With his plate-loaded barbell, Alan Calvert didn't look to the past for answers. He brought Physical Culture forward. So did Mark Berry, Bob Hoffman, Peary Rader, and Arthur Jones. Thank goodness Stuart McRobert looked to improve and advance Physical Culture in 1989 with *Hardgainer*, or we'd only have drug magazines to read!

If I had a gun to my head and could only choose one of the two exercises, I'd do the overhead press. You don't have a gun to your head, so unless you're lazy or physically limited, do both exercises!

Q. *I've read some articles on the web that mention "barf buckets" when doing HIT-style workouts. I've never barfed when training. Am I working hard enough?*

A Forget about barfing. It's not a measurement of hard work. It means nothing. If you train hard and never puke, that's *great.* It means that you're smart and know your body. I hope you never puke while training. I wrote a few articles that were stories about certain individuals who happen to have the propensity to barf, but it's no measurement of hard work.

Most of my clients have never barfed, so don't get the wrong message. It's usually the younger clients who are just starting with me and want to go hard right from the start. They almost challenge me to push them. They usually underestimate the intensity and want me to push them hard when they really have no idea what they are getting into. They are not used to the intensity. After a few workouts, barfing rarely happens once they get used to training hard.

With older clients, barfing never happens because I'm *very* careful with them and force them to start slowly. Some people may have a propensity for barfing, so we have a bucket handy to avoid a mess. *But I don't want barfing to happen.* I consider it a mistake by the trainer/coach if he makes his client puke. Sometimes barfing happens by accident and can come on fast. The only reason that I have a bucket is 'just in case.' If someone needs a little more rest between sets or exercises to avoid puking, *I greatly encourage it.*

Q. *What are some methods you use to help your clients get maximum results?*

A. Once trainees have completed the initial conditioning phase and are able to complete the planned workout, my number one goal as coach is to get them through it. I would be hurting their training if I flattened them before all the training was completed at any given workout. Knocking someone out early in a workout is easy. The human body can take only so much. Any coach can flatten someone, but a good coach tries to get each trainee through the entire workout with hard work throughout. That's the challenge of coaching. If a trainee needs to lay down for a few minutes, that's okay, but I want him or her back up to finish the workout. I want to push him or her to the edge of the cliff but not over it until all the planned work is done.

Achieving this requires different techniques for different people. Some need an extra minute of rest at a few key points during the workout. Some need positive strokes, and some need to be yelled at. It depends on their personality and what motivates them. That's what you do as a coach. You find out what works for your clients as individuals.

Some trainees like or need a lot of shouting, and some don't. some need a goal drilled into their head. They need a target because they have trouble thinking in terms of "going to failure." I usually give such trainees a high number that would be hard to reach so they will go to failure by accident. But they need a number to target, so on purpose I give one that's too high.

Other people don't want to know the weight on the bar or have any knowledge of their previous best performances for reps, because this puts pressure on them. I lie a lot to these people. I'll tell them the wrong weight (usually that it's lighter) or not tell them the weight or reps until they are done. I frequently give them wrong information on purpose so they won't know what to expect. My goal with them is to take the pressure off. Some people respond well to pressure and some don't. It's the coach's job to learn what motivates each athlete. The coach should still push to get the best out of each trainee but use a different mental technique in doing so, when necessary.

Exercise sequence is another big factor in the success of many of my clients. In my opinion, most people will not do justice to the rest of their workout if they train legs first, especially with a moderate volume workout. Don't get hung up on absolute rules such as "always work larger muscles first." That's just a general guidelines.

There are other less popular theories of exercise sequence such as pre-exhaustion, which is usually the opposite of working the largest muscles first. And there's the bodybuilding philosophy of working the weakest bodypart first or working first the parts of the physique that need the most improvement in order to bring about symmetry. Exercise sequence for me boils down to *performance* strategy.

You'll usually do better at what you do first or at the beginning of a workout, but you don't want to do anything first that greatly alters (or ends) the rest of the workout. The philosophy of working the larger muscles first is good in theory and in practice for many people—mainly if your workouts are short, i.e. 20 minutes or so—but for some trainees, especially those who do more volume and sets to failure, it's a disaster.

When training for general fitness or a powerlifting-type routine with lots of rest and low reps, it's easy to train the larger muscles first. Performance strategy depends on your style of training. For really intensive training with minimal rest between sets, just one all-out set to failure of deadlifts or squats at the beginning could end the entire workout for many trainees.

This is especially true when doing multiple sets. Remember that may "larger muscles first" advocates (who train in a high-intensity fashion) usually do just one set to failure per exercise. Single-set training to failure is tough, but multiple sets to failure for a lower-body exercise is suicidal for many people if done at the beginning of a workout. If you do multiple sets and feel impaired after doing legs first in a workout, try doing legs at the end of your workout. You're also supposed to *enjoy* your training. If you like to do legs first, fine. But if it's agony for you and impairs the rest of your workout, don't do it.

I don't want my clients to do just squats and then be done. I also don't want them to be impaired to the point that they are weak in upper-body exercises because they are wiped out. I've found that upper-body exercises don't affect the lower-body exercises nearly as much as vice versa. Many if not most of my clients do their squats, deadlifts and leg presses after everything else is done. That way, if they are KOed, it's the end of the workout and everything else has already been done so nothing gets sacrificed.

Another rule I follow is using an equal number of pushing and pulling exercises at each workout. I usually perform a pushing and a pulling exercise for the horizontal and vertical planes for the upper body at each workout and use a form of squat as a lower-body push and a form of deadlift as a lower-body pull. We also use the Hammer Leg Press as an alternative leg movement. Pushing and pulling for the horizontal and vertical planes for the upper body at each workout may be too much for some people. They may respond better to training the horizontal and vertical planes just once a week each. For some advanced trainees, I may use the deadlift and leg press in the same workout.

It's a good idea to alternate the pushing and pulling exercises so there's built-in recovery between exercises even though you're not actually resting. You'll lose too much strength if you do multiple pushing or pulling exercises back to back, e.g., overhead press followed by the bench press.

I usually have my clients perform three exercises in a row with no rest between sets and then have them take a minutes or two of rest. It's a push-pull-legs sequence. We do two sets and then do a second round of this format but with different exercises. Usually in the first round we substitute an isolation exercise, e.g., two-inch thick-bar curls, for the leg movement and do the leg movement only on the second round. Here's an illustration:

First round
First set
   Bench press
   Row
   Thick-bar curl
Rest
   Neck
   Grip

Second set
   Bench press
   Row
   Thick-bar curl
Rest
   Abs

306

Now the workout is half over.

Second round
    Overhead press
    Pulldown
    Squat
    Rest 2-3 minutes
    Neck, abs, *or* grip

Then we repeat the second round for a second set. Then it's workout over. All of that is takes about one hour or a little less.

I'm a big believer in employing a change-of--pace day once in a while. Mixing up your training is helpful and makes exercise fun. It's also smart because it motivates. When you establish certain traditions on certain days of the month or year, you really look forward to those special days and get motivated. Motivation is the key to training success. Slow days of various speeds, breakdown sets day, 50s day, are just some examples of things you can do for a change of pace.

Finishers done periodically at the end of the workout (for some able-bodied people) are also helpful to create camaraderie and motivation. Motivation is developed by the sandbag, Atomic Stones, and farmer's walk. In my experience, some of the younger guys will "kill" themselves on these finishers and greatly look forward to them. I've had people drive five hours to Washington, DC, mainly for the sandbag or farmer's walk. That's all they talked about. I'm all for whatever works to inspire greater effort.

When you mix up your training, remember that this strategy is still part of the overall plan—it's not haphazard. The planned change-of-pace days still incorporate the basic WST principles but are performed in a different manner.

Red Wine and HDL Levels

Previously, I noted some factors that raise blood HDL—i.e., the so-called "good" cholesterol as against the LDL, the so-called "bad" cholesterol—as mainly exercise and time released niacin.

There's another popular way to raise HDL besides niacin and exercise—red wine, but *only* one or two glasses per day, not more than that. Some people use this possible benefit of moderate wine consumption as an excuse to drink more than two glasses, which isn't helpful.

BOB WHELAN'S Q&A

May 2003

Dr. Ken and the Press/Bench Press

Dr. Ken is a class act, and I appreciate the fact that he contacted me before he had submitted his article to *Hardgainer* so I could respond in the same issue if I wanted to. We discussed the topic; he told me his opinion and I told him mine. No two people agree on everything. Ken and I agree on probably 95% of training topics, and we mostly agree on the issue of the press. We both feel this is only a minor area of disagreement, but it's valuable for readers to see different views.

I have a tremendous amount of respect for Dr. Ken and value his opinion greatly. Over the years, I've called him for advice many times. Whether it be about the quality of certain equipment, getting a new machine, how to contact an individual, or information on any sort of training topic, I've gone to Ken and will continue to do so.

We agree that the bench press is overrated greatly by most trainees and shouldn't be the lift to "base your ego on," as it is now for many trainees. I've written about this for years, as has Ken. We agree that overtraining and improper use of the bench press can cause the injuries that Ken described. We also agree that if we had a gun to our heads and had to choose one exercise, we'd pick the overhead press. I said that in the previous chapter.

I just don't agree that a horizontal push (usually the bench press) should be left out of a balanced program. I also feel that "proper use" of the bench press—i.e., not overtraining it—is productive and should be done by those who use it as their horizontal push. You can overtrain any lift, including the bench press. There's another factor to consider: I've had many trainees who can't overhead press because of compression on their spines. For them, the horizontal push increases in importance.

I've always believed in balanced training. When Dan Riley was the Strength Coach of the Washington Redskins and was in the local DC area, I talked to him a lot. I was greatly influenced by his *planes of motion* philosophy. He uses more planes of motion than I do, but I devised a program of *limited* balanced planes to suit my more abbreviated training philosophy.

I believe that a horizontal push *and* a vertical push are better than just doing one of them in a training program. That's it, in a nutshell. I guess we could also agree that a "safer horizontal push," such as the Hammer Chest Press or Southern Xercise's Horizontal True-Press (which is what we use at WST most of the time), could be used more productively by people who are bothered by the bench press.

Q. *I've heard that you have a Hammer Strength Four-Way Neck Machine at WST. What do you think of the machine, and how do you use it?*

A. I've always believed in working the neck area. I bought the four-way neck machine about six years ago. The machine is great, and I've been spoiled by it. After spending time with this unit, it would be hard for me to go back to the stuff I used formerly. It would be like going back to the horse and buggy after having had a car. We used to use the neck harness and manual resistance, which can get the job done. The side-to-side motion with the neck harness isn't great, though, and even the forward motion can cause some discomfort depending on how it's done. For manual resistance neck work, you must rely on the skill of the person providing the resistance. It can be good or bad depending on how competent the individual is at providing the resistance.

These problems are pretty much solved with the machine. You can get complete four-way motion in a safe and controlled fashion. It's hard to mess this up providing you use the machine sensibly. Monitoring progression is a lot easier because you can have a definite target and form is controlled. With manual resistance, though, the resistance can't be incrementally progressive. What you get a lot of the time with manual resistance is a lot of hard work, but not necessarily a good form of strength training. Monitoring load progression is the key element of successful strength training. Hard work alone will just burn a lot of calories and make you tired.

The way we use the machine is by working each part of the neck once per week. We normally do the front and back of the neck on one training day and the sides on the other workout day (in a twice-per-week training format). If I see a trainee only one per week—since he trains on his own once per week—we usually do all four motions on the day he trains with me, and he does no neck work in his other workout.

You must start out light and be patient when working your neck. Having a sore neck isn't like having sore biceps. I've strained my neck in the past and felt it every waking hour and couldn't sleep well, either. Avoid getting a sore neck. Go extremely light the first few times using this machine. You have to get used to it and feel comfortable with the motions. It's not uncommon for me to start someone with no more than just ten pounds to see how he/she reacts to the first neck workout.

When I first got the machine, I used a regular speed of motion. The longer I have a certain machine, the more I learn about it. I tweak it and find flaws and ways to improve what I'm doing. I now put neck work into a special category. For the last three or four years we've done neck work at about 8-10 seconds for the positive phase and a further 8-10 seconds or so for the negative phase. I'm not, however, strict on the exact count as long as the reps are done slowly and under control. I feel this is safer for the neck area and prevents rapid movement under load and a possible whiplash effect on the neck/upper spine. Seat positioning and head placement in the head pad are very important. I'll provide some tips for each movement.

Front Motion

This, I feel, is potentially the most dangerous neck movement, especially the negative or eccentric part. I know some coaches who won't do the front motion because they consider it too dangerous. This is partly because of the whiplash effect (acceleration/ deceleration) that can take place due to not pausing at the midpoint and not lowering the resistance under control. But even if you go slowly with a lot of weight, the negative/ eccentric motion is potentially dangerous and can strain the connecting muscle at the base of the skull.

The front motion can be used, however, if you're extremely careful, use a *slow* and *controlled* speed throughout each rep, start with a *very light weight*, and avoid any sort of bouncing or rapid change between the positive and negative motions. The change in direction at the midpoint of the rep from concentric to eccentric motion must be done in a slow and smooth way.

When doing the front movement, make sure that the face pad fits properly—like a baseball catcher's mask. Don't have it too low so that you're pushing with your jaw or too high so you're pushing with your forehead. It should be evenly distributed on your entire face. Face positioning like a catcher's mask is the critical element to determine where to adjust the seat for you.

The seat position adjustment is determined by torso length, not your overall height, so be extra careful to get the seat positioning right for you, and mark the pin position in your training log to keep it right every workout. Making a mistake in seat placement can cause neck strain.

I have the client hold the handles and have the torso leaning forward slightly. I use a controlled 8-10/8-10 second speed on all four motions of the machine, not just the front motion. We also have a one-second pause at the midpoint transition of the rep.

I slowly, I repeat *slowly*, increase poundage on the neck machine as strength increase permits. We aim to get five slow reps per set before there's any weight increase. Neck poundage progression is purposely retarded at WST to avoid neck strain. We make progress, but a lot slower than for other exercises. You can't be too careful when working the neck, especially the front part.

Rear Motion

You can use more weight on the rear motion than the front one, as the trapezius muscles of the upper back and neck are stronger than the frontal neck musculature. Since you can't bend your neck far backwards from an upright starting position, the key element for increasing the range of motion for the rear movement is correct positioning. Sit in the seat in a way that allows your chin to come down into your upper chest at the start and end of each rep. in other words, *don't* start and finish each rep from the upright position, but take great care not to overextend the range of motion.

Keep your shoulders and butt back so you can get your chin closer to your chest in a smooth and easy motion. If it's a strain to do this, you're not in a good seat position. Put no weight on the machine and experiment to find the best seat positioning for you. (Make a note of the seat setting in your training log.) Only then should you start to increase resistance slowly and carefully.

Make sure you have a solid heat fit on the head pad. Again, we use five slow 8-10/8-10 second reps.

Side-to-Side Motion

Be sure to plant your feet well apart, as this helps you to push sideways easier. Make sure the center of your head is against the pad. Many people have restricted movement in the lateral motion because they have the pad too high on their heads. Apply the same rules of rep speed, and great care in general, as with the other motions.

The prime movers of the front and lateral neck motions are the sternocleidomastoid muscles of the front part of the neck. These are smaller and weaker than the trapezius muscles of the upper back and neck. Balanced neck training doesn't mean that you'll use the same poundage in the front and side motions as you do in the back motion. The back motion can employ a higher poundage than the other motions. But regardless of which motion you do, only use a weight you can handle properly in a smooth and slow form.

Q. *I've heard that you have a great collection of ole Iron Game books and magazines. Which items in your collection are your favorites?*

A. I have a good collection, but it's not in the league of the top collectors. There are many people who are seriously into collecting and have much larger collections than I do. I started casually collecting (or saving) old magazines and books when I was a kid, but I didn't put much effort into it. I was too busy training.

I remember giving away some old books to friends in the military. I had an old Professor Titus course from the early 1900s that a friend found in his attic and gave to me. I don't have it any more and don't know what I did with it. I would love to have it now! I lost many items when moving.

It wasn't until I became friends with Osmo Kiiha that I began to take collecting seriously. I rounded up all my old stuff and took better care of it. Osmo introduced me to several prominent collectors, and I bought a few things at a time. Collecting is like training—just keep at it. Besides Osmo (who sold me a lot of stuff), I also bought items from Bill Hinbern, Angelo Iupsa, Howard Havener, Bob Adams, and Jeff Gretz. (Most of these guys are listed on my website.

I was lucky and got *Super Strength* by Alan Calvert (1924) right away but it took me about five years to get *The Key to Might & Muscle* by George Jowett (1926). Collecting is a lot of luck as some things fall into your lap almost by accident. If you just keep looking, you can find a lot of great items.

One of my favorite items is *How to Get Strong and How to Stay So* by William Blaikie (1979). This is the book that inspired many of the old timers like MacFadden and Calvert. Another favorite, Calvert's *Super Strength*, may be the most influential book ever written in strength training. Almost every training book thereafter has roots in *Super Strength.*

Jan Dellinger told me at a Capital City Strength Clinic that when he shared an office with John Grimek for several years at York Barbell Company, the only book that John always kept on the shelf above his desk was a copy of Calvert's *Super Strength*, even though Bob Hoffman didn't like the copy being kept in Grimek's office.

Calvert founded Milo Barbell Company (1902) and *Strength* magazine (1914). We all owe Calvert a lot of gratitude for what he did for moving strength training into the modern age. He was an Iron Game giant and put the *adjustable* barbell into the hands of the masses. He made it possible to progress by adding *incremental* weight (without having to own a junkyard full of items). Calvert is probably the most underappreciated and underrated individual in the history of Physical Culture. He may have been the greatest ever but gets little recognition by most people.

I like some books because they are different or strange, e.g., Hoffman's *I Remember the Last War* and *Your Sex Life Before Marriage.* I have just about every book Hoffman wrote. My favorite Hoffman book (to actually read cover to cover) is *How to be Strong, Healthy and Happy.*

I have about 50 books and booklets by Bernarr MacFadden, whom I greatly admire as a pioneer. I have several Mark Berry, George Jowett, and Earle Leiderman books, courses, and booklets. I have a lot of reprinted old courses and books from Bill Hinbern and a good collection of old magazines including *Physical Culture, The Strongman, Strength, Strength & Health*, and *Iron Man*.

Bob Adams recently sold me many *Strength & Health* from the 1930s, 40s, and 50s, in mint condition. I have the first four years of *Muscular Development* in mint condition and many afterwards. I especially treasure the first issue of *Muscular Development*, January 1964, with Grimek on the cover.

Probably my favorite items are in my Sandow collection. Jeff Gretz had several Sandow items and for years he would be on the verge of selling them to me but then would change his mind. Several years ago, I gave Jeff a big offer right before Christmas—when he needed money for presents. It worked! I got **Sandow's** *System of Physical Training* (first edition), *Life is Movement* (first and second editions), *Strength & How to Obtain It* (first, second, and revised editions), and **Sandow's Magazine of Physical Culture**, Volume 8, 1902 January-June, bound. Probably the most valuable piece I got is a rare Sandow postal instruction mail order course from 1906 and that I keep in plastic.

BOB WHELAN'S Q&A

July 2003

Q. *I don't seem to be making progress of late and believe that I* *may be overtraining. I work out twice a week but train each* *bodypart once per week. My workouts usually last about 30* *minutes. Am I doing too much? Should I cut back to just one* *workout per week?*

A. Let me first address the issue of "real overtraining." When I first started lifting, in the mid-1960s, I would train for two hours or longer at each workout. I would usually train on a four-day split but also tried three workouts per week, and even five and six workouts per week, but usually did the four. It was normal for me. Of course, I felt tired and sore, and was *definitely* overtraining, but I didn't know any better. But I still made good progress because I was young at the time and my recovery system was at its peak.

After several years of reading what Peary Rader had to say about overtraining, I finally cut back to two whole-body workouts per week. It took me a while before I did it, though. I felt like I was loafing and barely training, only doing two workouts per week. But lo and behold, I got a *lot stronger!* The tired feeling and aching joints went away, sticking points vanished, and poundages went way, way up! I was sold and have been an advocate of "abbreviated" training ever since. But true abbreviated training isn't undertraining (or almost nontraining).

What's meant by "abbreviated"? It doesn't mean the same thing as "the minimum." The idea that we should try to do the minimum amount of work to get the job done is wrong. Aiming and searching for the minimum, like there's a reward for it, is what gets people on the path to failing and underachievement. The right amount of training is what you should be aiming for, and that doesn't necessarily mean less training. It's almost become a sacred tradition in drug-free training circles to always aim for less training.

On suspicion of a training problem, the usual automatic target is overtraining, and it's true in many cases. But there are many drug-free people who are not getting the results they want because they are *barely* training. They are not training enough!

If you were training two or more hours per workout, four or more days per week, I would say you were overtraining and would advise you to cut way back. I would definitely not cut back *your* (the questioner's) training. When you're already on an abbreviated program, cutting back even more is not the answer. It turns abbreviated training into undertraining. I would keep training twice every 7-10 days and train the whole body each workout.

I think this particular question may be a mental toughness (or mental negativity) issue more than a physical issue. Work on your attitude. Read the "Mind Strength" section at NaturalStrength.com.

Evaluate your diet—always eat breakfast and get enough protein. And evaluate your sleep and other habits such as alcohol consumption. Do you enjoy training? If so, spend more time training but without overdoing it. Try working each major muscle group every workout in true whole-body format. If you're already training just twice a week and less than an hour at each workout, it would be hard to convince me that you're overtraining.

Q. *What do you think of the pullover as an exercise? Is it a pushing or pulling movement? How do you use it at WST?*

A. I've always included some form of pullover in my own training program. I have a relationship with the exercise lasting over 35 years. There are two main types of pullovers. The first and most common is the muscle-building type, and the second is the

318

"breathing" type.

The breathing pullover employs a very light barbell and straight arms. The goal here isn't poundage progression but stretching and deep breathing, with the goal to expand the rib cage. It's controversial as to whether you believe rib cage expansion is possible through this exercise. Physical Culture tradition and folklore say it is. Many in the scientific community say it isn't possible. All I can say is that, as a youngster, when I first started training and through high school, this is the main type of pullover I did. I have a deep and huge rib cage for my height. I'll never know for sure if it was the breathing pullovers that were responsible, but let's just say they did me no harm. The breathing pullover is especially productive in the early years of training.

The rest of this segment will focus on the muscle-building type of pullover where the elbows are bent and the goal is progression and muscle building. (The machine pullover is always the muscle-building type.) this is probably the most common type of pullover today.

On the muscle-building pullover, for decades I used an ez-curl bar lying over the edge of a bench and got great results. I've only used the machine version for the last several years. You can get great results with either free weights or a machine as long as you do the exercise right.

When using a bar, be careful not to hyperextend your shoulders by going down too far—especially when you first start doing the exercise. You have to get used to it, and you'll develop more flexibility after several workouts. Also, be careful not to try one too many reps, as you can give yourself a black eye and bruised face by dragging the bar over your face on the final "one too many" rep.

I remember when I was in my twenties, I used to do pullovers on Friday. I would always go all out on them and had to turn my head sideways so as not to hit my nose, and then just scrape my face

319

with the bar o the last rep. I gave myself a few black eyes, and it looked like I'd gotten into a fight or something when I'd go out with my friends on Friday nights. People wouldn't believe it was from lifting weights!

This is one of the few exercises where I prefer a machine to a barbell. If you have access to a Hammer Strength type of pullover, I would recommend it over using a barbell for safety reasons. In addition to keeping you from dragging the bar across your face, the machine pullover also limits the range of motion better. Even with the machine pullover, be careful not to use an excessive range of motion.

As far as being a pushing or pulling exercise, the machine version is both, but I put it in the pulling category when I devise my workouts. The beginning part of the exercise, when the weight is raised from the bottom position, starts out as a pulling exercise and stays so for most of the range of motion. During the last part of the concentric movement, the pushing muscles, mainly triceps and pectorals, come into play when pushing the crossbar to the waist area.

Arthur Jones coined the pullover as "the upper-body squat" because it works almost every major muscle group in the upper body.

It makes a significant difference if you get the crossbar to the waist and hold it there for a second before entering the eccentric phase of the motion. Near the end of the set, you may not be able to come all the way down, so still give it a full second ("one-one-thousand") hold at the furthest point closest to your waist. Lower the weight slowly on the eccentric phase and don't bounce off the bottom if you can go all the way down for a full range of motion.

Q. *I recently cut carbohydrates out of my diet. Could this be why I now feel weak and tired when I try to train hard?*

A. Yes, this is *exactly* why. Cutting down on "wasted calorie carbs" like white flour products and junk food is a good thing. Cutting out the fast-burning simple carbohydrates such as sugar is great, but *don't* cut out the good carbs.

The good carbs are the complex ones found in fruit, vegetables, whole grains, and legumes. To me, anyone on a zero-carb diet is just showing ignorance. What fuel do you think your brain uses? Have you ever heard of the Krebs cycle, energy systems, ATP or fast twitch muscle fibers?

When you strength train, you burn carbohydrates as fuel. Your body can't compensate for poor fuel. If you're out of gas and are inadequately fueled, you're not capable of training hard and are doomed to fail. You can get all the rest and recovery you want, be mentally focused, and eat lots of protein, but you'll still feel weak and tired if you don't have enough glycogen storage in your muscles and liver. You'll not make it through your workout. Complex carbohydrates are essential to your training success. Don't be fooled by the quackery.

If you don't believe me or need more than common sense information, go to a registered dietician for advice. Never go to a health food store for advice. That is the last place you should be asking questions. All you'll likely get there are minimum-wage employees who recite the manufacturers' sales pitches.

Don't read the mainstream megahype drug-infested muscle mags for advice, either. Don't go to (most) gyms for advice on nutrition either, as they are no better and will try to sell you pills and powders—most of which are a waste of money, or worse. Don't ask bodybuilders for nutritional advice; don't ask your friends for advice on nutrition; don't ask your co-workers for nutritional advice. See a registered dietician. I think you get it now!

Q. *what do you think of working calves?*

A. I'm never going to say not to work a specific muscle. Ideally, calves should be worked like every other muscle. In the real world, due to time constraints and other reasons or excuses, some exercises get sacrificed, and that has been the case for me the last few years with calves. I used to work calves regularly for decades but then fell into the habit of leaving them out due to lack of time. I rationalized that they were getting enough indirect work from squats, leg presses, and deadlifts. I recently thought about this and had a change of heart. It only takes a few minutes to add calf work to your routine. I made a calf raise platform from some 2x4s. It works great for standing calf raises on the Tru-Squat.

We all can find ways to improve our training programs. If you're not doing calf work, find the time. It only takes a few minutes, and there really is no good excuse not to work your calves.

Q. *I'm starting a home gym in my basement. I want bang for my buck. What equipment would you recommend on a limited budget?*

A. The first three things I would recommend are a good Olympic bar and plates, a good power rack, and a good *adjustable* heavy-duty bench. Even if this is all that you buy, it's enough to get the job done well. You really don't need any more equipment than this.

It's better to buy quality than buy cheap. I would get an Olympic bar and plates from York, Eleiko, Ivanko, or Leoko. Naturalstrength.com has links to all of them in the resource/link section.

The power rack and bench should be heavy duty. You need

strength for safety. Make sure the bench is sturdy and can be adjusted on both ends. Raising the seat end keeps you from sliding on incline presses and seated military presses. You can do your whole workout in the power rack: bench presses, incline presses, military presses, Olympic lifts, shrugs, deadlifts, squats, etc. Some racks even have a bar across the top you can use for chins. Shop around for quality equipment and a good price.

Q. *Out of the various training methods, e.g., HIT, Dino, SuperSlow, and NSCA, which do you recommend?*

A. I recommend and use *progressive strength training.* Period. I like being free to use my own mind to use whatever works for me. I don't like being pigeon-holed into a philosophy or part of a group that has limited views on training. Free yourself from that and use your own instincts. No one in these camps invented the actual exercises. There are productive exercises and methods in each camp, but they are grouped together by false boundaries.

As I've said before, I see myself as a tradesman with a shed full of tools. I want the option to use whatever tool I see fit, not just a pre-selected few of them. Who says you can't use singles, machines, barbells, odd objects, and slow training in your program? You can use whatever works best for your goals and physical capacity or for the individual you're training. I've done workouts that had low reps with barbells in pyramid style in part of it, slow training on a machine in one exercise, sets to failure on a few exercises, and then finish with odd objects. I'd just call it natural, hard and progressive strength training. As long as what you do makes sense and you enjoy it, that's the key. Just be sure it's safe and productive and helps you meet your goals.

Q. *I usually train three times a week on a handful of basic compound exercises. I tried cutting down to twice a week but I lost strength. Why?*

A. Total weekly volume and intensity usually determines which works better, two or three workouts per week. If you train hard three times per week, you'll probably have shorter workouts (or otherwise you could overtrain) and use the three workouts to balance out your program. If you switch over to two workouts, make the workouts higher volume and full body, or you may end up undertraining.

If you're truly training hard in a balanced whole body format, there's no way you would lose strength while training twice per week. It's *how* you train that determines whether three or two times per week works better. Both can work.

The old heavy-light-medium format will work while training the whole body three times a week, but that way, you're training heavy/hard only once per week, which is actually *less* work overall in my opinion. If you train like we do at WST, with a balanced whole-body routine—including neck, abs, calves, and grip, for one hour of training with little rest between sets and exercises—and train heavily and hard with mostly compound exercises, you'd be physically incapable of handling more than two workouts per week.

BOB WHELAN'S Q&A

September 2003

Q. *Many of my friends train different muscles on different days.* They claim this is *"more advanced"* than training the whole body *each workout. Is this true?*

A. No, it's the opposite. Bodypart training has been around for several decades. It really became a lot more popular since the inception of drug use over 40 years ago. This philosophy is pushed by the megahype, drug-infested magazines. If someone is a natural lifter and follows that type of training, he's not more advanced but probably a beginner who's being sucked in by the drug-pimping promoters. The more advanced and knowledgeable he gets or the more money he wastes on supplements (which is the lie of why these bodypart programs are supposed to work when it's really the drugs), or the overall lack of progress he gets, the more likely the trainee will come to his senses and train only two or three times per week. This assumes that the trainee's true intent is to stay natural without using steroids.

Bodypart training and natural training usually don't mix. Most people who train bodyparts (not the whole body) confuse "training" with "going to the gym." They somehow believe that by going into a building called the gym, they will get bigger and stronger. They rarely talk about poundages on heavy squats and other basic lifts or how hard they work, but instead talk about time spent in a building. They brag about how long they are "in the gym" and how often they "go to the gym." They believe that by training bodyparts, and thus spending more time "in the gym," they will get better results. They are usually unsophisticated beginners. Most guys who "go to the gym" usually spend more time talking an socializing at the water fountain than they do training. That's why they are there for three hours! They take a ten-minute rest between sets and usually bench press with several other people. Their bench press workout alone takes 30 to 40 minutes. These guys rarely break a sweat!

It's hard to train bodyparts without overtraining from muscle overlap. You can't put the major, multi-joint exercises into neat, separate categories. The bench press, for example, doesn't hit just the chest but front delts and triceps. The machine pullover, termed the "upper-body squat," works almost every muscle in the upper body. What category do you put it in?

If you train hard five or six days per week, you'll overtrain. Those who train five or six days per week (and don't overtrain) are either on drugs or are not working hard. They take long rests between sets and the workout is filled with easy exercises such as triceps kickbacks, cable cross-overs, lateral raises, flyes, and leg extensions. They don't do heavy squats, deadlifts, chins, rows, military presses, etc.

You don't get the thick, muscular look unless you do the heavy compound exercises—the ones that require lots of recovery time for natural guys. Dr. Ken stated that people who do bodypart training look like they are a "collection of bodyparts" that don't seem to fit together.

The "look of power" is developed from using whole-body, compound-movement programs. That means thickness in the back, traps, glutes, legs, neck, and whole body, not just the arms and chest. If people only know that you "lift weights" when you have a tank top on, you don't have the look of power. The look of power can't be hidden. It has nothing to do with cuts or definition but size and thickness. If you have the look of power, then no matter what oversize, baggy sweatshirt you have on, you'll still look powerful.

It's no accident that bodypart training and drug use grew together and are from the same roots. Most people get innocently sucked into bodypart training without realizing it. The truth is that "bodypart routines" are usually drug or wimp routines and aren't effective for most drug-free trainees.

326

One alternative to two- and three-day whole-body routines would be a four-day split program if properly divided into upper body for two days and lower body for the other two days. This can be beneficial only for some young, enthusiastic trainees with good genetics for training. It could also be done in a push/pull format with good results. This is not bodypart training. The focus is still on the basic compound movements. I've had success with these four-day splits but only for a limited group of trainees. It's not for hard gainers or any middle-aged or older trainee.

For most natural lifters, I feel that whole-body training is the best road to take and typically just two times per week. The general recommendation I've mentioned before is two hard workouts every seven to ten days, depending on individual recovery ability.

If you train heavy, hard, and naturally, you'll learn what works and realize that the most advanced way to train for natural lifters is the whole-body program focusing on the basic exercises. This is as advanced as you can get, but many people are too ignorant to see the truth.

Q. *What's the best way to spot someone who's squatting?*

A. I get behind the trainee and squat right down with him or her. If they need just a little help, I usually tuck my hands under their elbows and pull them up. If they are really getting crushed, I ram my arms under their armpits and pull them up. I think this is better than having a guy at each end of the bar where the bar can be lifted up unevenly and cause injury to the lifter. In addition, unless in a powerlifting meet, you should always squat in a power rack with the pins set so that you can safely dump the weight if you have to, even if you have no spotter.

Q. *I've read a lot about the push-pull-legs-rest-isolation sequence*

you use, and I want to hear more. Please explain the exercise sequencing that you use at WST.

A. I've developed my own pattern of sequence that I call the WST sequence. My goal is to get the most amount of work done per unit of time without making the workout into an endurance or cardiovascular type session. At WST we focus on strength, or lifting as heavily as possible. Usually, that can't be done unless you get a lot of rest between sets. Using the WST sequence, that's all changed.

The traditional way is to train the larger muscles first and complete all sets and rest periods for a given exercise before moving to the next movement. I devised a system that manipulates the sequence to allow a lot of rest for the prime movers for optimum strength but without standing around resting and wasting time between sets.

There are few absolute rules in strength training, and this applies to exercise sequence, too. Working the largest muscles first can be a good rule for some, depending on how they train, but for others, it's a disaster. It's all about how you train.

I alternate pushing and pulling exercises and follow them with a major leg movement in the second half of the workout. Usually, in the first half of the workout, we'll do a major push or pull followed by something like shrugs or curls, then do neck, one grip exercise, and an about exercise. Then, following a short rest, we'd repeat the sequence but this time with a different grip exercise. For the neck, we do rearward and forward motions one workout and side-to-side flexion the other workout.

The second round of exercises in the second half of the workout would be a push-pull-legs-rest-isolation format. An example would be military presses followed by pulldowns followed by squats, then a rest, then calves, and then we'd repeat for a second set. For some young, well conditioned, enthusiastic trainees, we'll do the push-pull-legs sequence in both halves of the workout.

Working legs first is great if you like to do it that way, but it's very tough. Some people, especially beginners, would be better off doing legs at the end of their planned workouts. I know, from experience, that people don't like paying for an hour's workout if they train (doing legs first) for only a few minutes and then spend the rest of the workout wiped out and incapable of doing much if anything else.

As I've said before, training hard should be everyone's goal, but if you knock yourself out early and don't finish all the planned work, you're selling yourself short. Design your program in a manner that makes you enjoy your training and enables you to finish all the planned work.

Alternate pushing and pulling exercises to give your muscles additional time to rest, even though your actual rest between exercises is minimal. While your pushing muscles are working, your pulling muscles are getting a rest. I usually do three exercises in a row and then give a minute's rest, but I give a longer rest after squats, deadlifts, or leg presses.

I'm creative and manipulate exercise sequence to help the client (or me) finish all the work without wasting time. I don't always do it exactly the same way and have given you just some rough examples of how I often do it. Use your own instincts as I do. If a client is really wiped out after a heavy sets of squats, for example, I may give him a longer rest of four minutes or more and then follow this with a longer series of easier exercises such as calf, grip, or about work to help his recovery.

Q. *What do you mean by "controlled failure"?*

A. At WST we usually do two works sets per exercise each workout, so I devised a way to make it productive for strength with higher volume but while still incorporating a going-to-failure philosophy. Controlled failure means that you control the first set and don't allow reps to go beyond the goal on the set. If the goal of the set is to get eight reps, you don't get more than eight on the first set. You stop at eight even if you can do more. But on the second set, you go to all-out failure regardless of rep count. If you do eight or more reps on the second set, using perfect form, you progress to a heavier weight next time.

Using this method, you don't waste strength and shoot your whole wad on the first set but save strength for the second set, to progress. You get the conditioning and neurological pathway/motor learning benefits of doing multiple sets and get the benefits of going to failure, too.

Q. *What feats of strength do you respect most of all?*

A. I've come to respect feats of strength with a regular barbell more and more over the last ten years or so. In the early 1990s, when odd objects were new on the scene, I was temporarily enchanted with seeing them lifted. Upon further review and reflection, I've now gone back to being most impressed by the basic barbell lifts. With the barbell lifts, you know what you're seeing, and there's little chance for illusion or trickery. Many times, with odd objects, people are more enchanted with the object than the actual poundage lifted. I think sometimes people can use odd objects to hide a strength deficiency, as it's harder to judge what they can really lift. You're also more likely to cut them slack due to the supposed awkwardness of the object and assume they could lift more if it was a balanced barbell. This assumption is probably not true most of the time. It looks cool to see a log lifted, but it's hard to judge unless you really know how much it weighs. It may even have chains on it, which also looks cool, but looking cool has no bearing on my appreciation of a feat of strength.

It's the same with some trainees who specialize on grip work and can close the #3 gripper, which is great, but then they think they are full-fledged strongmen when they can't squat 400 or bench press 275.

This is just my personal opinion, and I appreciate all feats of strength, but the guy who lifts the heavy barbell is easier to judge for whole-body strength and most likely to be the real deal.

Q. *What do you do for grip work training at WST, and how do you define grip work?*

A. There aren't many places that do as much grip work on a consistent basis as we do at WST. We do some form of grip work (and usually more than one) at every workout. Grip work means working your hands, which have to be strong to hold the barbell in order to get your whole body strong. The real purpose of grip work is to enable you to build whole-body strength. The grip is the weakest link in many trainees' chain.

Grip work builds the muscles and strengthens the connective tissues of the wrists, forearms, and hands.

I have two manual wrist rollers (thin and thick handles), a wrist roller machine, two pairs of custom thick handles to put on my Hammer Strength and Southern Xercise machines (that I can pop on and off when I choose), and several thick bars from 1-3/4 to 3 inches (though I rarely use anything over two inches now). I have a plate-loading crushing machine, IronMind's Titan's Telegraph Key for working individual digits, a Weaver stick, two-inch-thick handled dumbbells, and plates for pinching.

Few trainees understand the importance of grip work. I believe grip work is the litmus test for membership in the Physical Culture Fraternity. Here's what my late friend, coach Bob Hise II of Mav-Rik (who made the Weaver stick I use at WST) said: Everything starts with the hands. The first thing I do when I take on a new lifter is stress the importance of grip work. You'll never get close to doing your best without it. You need strong hands for every lift—even squatting."

I used to talk on the phone with Bob Hise frequently. He relayed a grip story about Steve Stanko. Stanko used to cut leather, making lifting belts for Bob Hoffman at York Barbell Company. One day, the knife slipped, and Stanko cut the palm of his hand, putting the knife almost all the way through it. He had a big meet scheduled a few days later, and everyone thought it would be impossible for him even to compete. It was a bad cut and required many stitches. He not only competed but won, setting a new national record in 1938. during the contest, according to Hise, the stitches broke and Stanko's hand was bleeding profusely. To "plug it up," he used a handful of chalk, and with his grip at half strength, still won! All the grip work Stanko had done paid off.

Our Iron Game heritage is filled with stories that feature the old-timers doing serious grip work. Take, for example, John Davis' clean of 308 pounds with a two-inch thick bar, Bob People's deadlift of 725-3/4 pounds with a pronated (not mixed) grip, Al Berger doing pinch grip chins from his two-inch-thick ceiling beams, Hermann Goerner's one-handed deadlift with 727-1/2 pounds, and Thomas Inch's one-handed deadlift of 172 pounds with a 2.47-inch thick-handled dumbbell. Warren Lincoln Travis, with just his right middle finger, lifted over 600 pounds. Vic Boff was a champion at the art of finger twisting, which was very popular years ago. John Grimek set the record in the Weaver stick lift, with 11 pounds with his right hand. Apollon's thick axle bar is still talked about today. Ian Bachelor could crush metal beer caps between his thumb and each of his four fingers. Notice that all the names I mentioned were also strong in their whole body, too, and did not train their grip only.

Serious grip work builds mental toughness, too. As a change of pace, try an entire workout using just thick bars and you'll see what I'm talking about. (You may have to do some of the pulling movements with lighter weights than usual, using a slow speed, or otherwise the bar will fall out of your hands.) The wrist roller is a must and can be easily made. Do it palms up and palms down. And include one or more of the Weaver/lever stick, finger pinching, and hand crushing exercises in your program, too.

IronMind sells everything dealing with grip work, including all types of devices to build both pinching and crushing strength. You don't have to train to be another Rich Sorin or John Brookfield to reap tremendous benefits from doing grip work. Consistency is the key. An extra ten minutes at the end of your workout or even less if you use a thick bar during your workout will reap tremendous benefits. *If you can't hold the bar, you can't lift it!*

Work into new grip exercises carefully and progressively. If you do too much too soon, you may get an injury.

BOB WHELAN'S Q&A

November 2003

Q. *Kettlebells seem to be the current fad, though an old idea. Some of the exercises I've seen demonstrated look to be high risk unless done with very light weights. What do you think about kettlebells?*

A. Kettlebells can be productive strength training tools for some trainees but are definitely not recommended for everybody (for *strength* training). Many individuals who employ kettlebells use them in extremely light poundages, which isn't strength training. This training is usually described and packaged by the marketers as fat burning, conditioning, or shaping. Kettlebells are currently popular used in this sort of way, especially with women.

This very light weight workout is done in a toning or cardio format. Kettlebells are safe and productive if used in this light toning way. If you want to look like a trim, wiry, fit, lean Russian commando, then go for it. If your goal is to build maximum muscular size and strength, (STRENGTH TRAINING) kettlebells aren't the best way to train, at least not when used in a light manner.

I'm devoting the rest of this answer to using kettlebells in a progressive, strength-training and muscle-building way—how the old, old-timers usually used them.

The best thing about kettlebells is that they can be fun and different. I have an antique one that is mostly for decoration at Whelan Strength Training, but I've used it on occasion. I also owned a pair of York handles and used them regularly in my very early training days. They seemed awkward and uncomfortable, though, and after my first few years of training, I rarely used the handles.

334

The York handles were made of black iron. They could be put on adjustable dumbbells to make the latter into kettlebells. They usually came with the York barbell sets. I think my first barbell set weighed 110 pounds, from York, which I got when I was 13. a pair of kettlebell handles came with it.

Now, when I'm bored with everything else, I might pull out the antique kettlebell and do some clean and presses with it, maybe once every few years. I find the kettlebell awkward and uncomfortable, and I don't like juggling movements, so I rarely use it. Kettlebells do make a change of pace, and for a different kind of workout. It really depends on whether you enjoy using them and if they are safe for you as they can be rough on the joints.

Kettlebells have a following of loyal users who swear by them but usually train with them TOO LIGHT. Kettlebells can be tremendous for grip, wrist, and forearm strength. I've heard from guys who like using them, who claim as much as an inch of growth in wrist size in only a few months, using nothing but kettlebells. The training can work, and many of the old, old-timers swore by them.

Using my own common sense, however, I believe that there must have been a good reason why training with heavy kettlebells (before their recent resurgence) fell out of favor over the last 70 years, just as odd-shaped objects did. If they were "all good all the time," they would have stayed as popular as barbells and dumbbells. What made them fall out of favor? I believe that progress and common sense made most of the old-timers favor a safer and more enjoyable way to get the job done than the old, old-timers used.

HEAVY and progressive use of kettlebells can be rough on the joints, especially if they are juggled, and need to be used very carefully. They can be an excellent conditioning tool for athletes involved in contact sports like kickboxing, wrestling, and football. They supposedly increase the ability of the body to absorb ballistic impact. The repetitive ballistic shock builds strong tendons and ligaments (for those who don't get injured in the process).

The ratio of injury potential versus the possible benefits seems high to me. I don't use kettlebells often and wouldn't use them with my own clients for liability reasons. I'm responsible for keeping my clients free of injury. If you're advanced, have a need for this sort of conditioning, and enjoy using kettlebells, then go for it, *but be careful.* In a way, kettlebells are similar to odd-shaped objects: They aren't *needed* but can be a productive addition for some trainees. But, they can also be disastrous for some trainees. If you use them, start light and *be careful.*

There are different types of kettlebells: shot-loaded, solid cast-iron, and steel with rotating handles. Each has its benefits. here are some basic exercises that are commonly done with kettlebells: one- and two-handed swing, press, curl, crucifix, repetition deadlifting, one-hand clean, one-hand snatch, Romanian deadlift. Wrist and forearm exercises are good with the kettlebells with the rotating handles.

Most people don't realize it, but York still sold kettlebell handles into the early 1980s. I believe they were the last company selling them until the recent resurgence. If you need to buy kettlebells, get in touch with Roger LaPointe at AtomicAthletic.com.

Q. *Please explain what exercises you use the Weaver stick for.*

A. I use the Weaver stick in the same way you would use a lever bar or sledge hammer. I use it usually once a week and hold it out straight with my arm parallel to the floor, and I try to keep from bending my elbow. Using just my wrist, I raise the handle 'til it's vertical, or the hanging weight comes up against the handle. Be careful not to smash your hand with the weight if the chain suspending the weight is short.

I go to failure with each hand and try to hold the stick or pipe further to the end away from the hanging weight. It gets harder the further to the end you hold on. You must choke up at first and grab the pipe near the middle. When you can use it easily, keeping your arm straight while holding at the very end of the stick or pipe, add weight. Use micro plates for progression, as a 2-1/2 pound plate increase with the Weaver stick would crush you.

Q. *Do you recommend the Swiss ball for ball squats, or anything else? If you do, please share your experiences.*

A. I'm not a big fan of it, but I also don't think that the use of any tool should be completely overlooked. The stability balls have been around a long time and, like all gadgets, have resurfaced with trendy names, colors, and a variety of different dimensions. They can be useful if used properly, but they can cause serious accidents if not used properly.

Rule #1: Don't try to make the ball into a bench. It's not a bench, and those who use it as a bench for heavy lifting are stupid.

Rule #2: Don't try to make the ball into the floor. The ball isn't the floor, and those who try to stand on it while lifting aren't just stupid but insane.

To use the ball to stand on or to replace a bench is, to me, colossal stupidity, but it's done frequently in commercial gyms under the guise of building balance and strength. I kid you not.

I've seen people in commercial gyms lie on their backs across Swiss balls while trying to bench press, sit on them to military press, and even try to squat while standing on them! I'm not joking. There are some people who believe that it's beneficial to do this, supposedly because it improves balance while strength training! They're crazy.

For certain abdominal exercises, wall and ball squats, and some light lifting support, they are great. Some are supposedly able to withstand up to 600 pounds of pressure. Base your selection according to your height, weight, and exercise intentions. They can be good training tools for some stretches and can be effective and useful in rehab.

Q. *In your writings, you've mentioned, for trainees who need to consume a great deal of nourishment, eating three balanced, high-protein meals (of food), drinking up to a gallon of milk a day, and eating two cans or tuna (or chicken or turkey) a day between meals. Is there a better way of getting enough protein? I use a protein powder—three small shakes a day give me an extra 70 grams of protein, on top of my three meals. Finding this level of protein for such a low cost, with minimal fat and calories, isn't just hard, it's impossible. Also, as it's in liquid form, I don't need to be hungry to get my protein foxes. What do you think?*

A. There's nothing wrong with using protein powder. I don't need it, however, because I like to eat, and I get 150 grams of protein a day without even trying. If you're the type who doesn't like to eat that much or has trouble eating enough, then it's better to have the powder than not get enough protein. I believe that most trainees don't need protein powder.

Two cans of turkey, chicken, or tuna give you about 90 grams of protein as snacks. One gallon of milk (it can be skim milk) gives you 120 grams of protein. You can do what I recommend just half-heartedly and still get 200 grams of protein a day. It's easy if you like to eat and have the appetite. If you're a finicky eater, take the powder.

But be sure you need this quantity of food and are training hard and progressively—otherwise you'll get fat.

Q. *Do you prefer adjustable grippers to fixed-resistance ones? Or, do you prefer the gripping machine to all forms of grippers? Either way, why?*

A. I prefer the weight-plate, adjustable crusher over the spring-type grippers for training. I have the numbered grippers to test my strength and occasionally use for training. My clients usually use the plate-loaded crusher for training. I believe that the plate-loaded crusher is better for training because it's easier to monitor progression.

If you use the spring-type grippers, it makes a big difference how you hold them. Hold the gripper high up on your hand, and have your hand as far down on the handles as possible. Your pinky finger should be at the very bottom, almost off the gripper. You lose leverage by holding it too close to the spring.

Q. *I have several old nagging injuries that seem to crop up just when things get going well. Is anyone out there doing slow training and noticing size increases? I've read some articles by Drew Israel about it. But wasn't Drew big before he used very slow training? I've dabbled in slow training but never stuck with it. Now, I'm wondering if I shouldn't give it a longer trial, hoping it would allow me to train without all these injuries messing up my progress. But, if it's not going to add size, then I need to find another alternative.*

A. Slow training can work well, especially if you have injuries. You'll gain strength in the slow format *if* you keep poundage progression a top priority and don't get obsessed with minor details of performance that retard poundage progression. Stick with the principles of abbreviated training, progression, etc., and train

339

slowly using a speed of five to ten seconds on each of the positive and negative phases of each rep, and your risk of injury should be minimized.

You'll gain strength in this style of training. Perhaps you'll gain some size, depending on your starting point and experience, and whether or not you're coming back from injury and atrophy.

Q. *How do you recommend strength training be combined with martial arts training without burning out in either?*

A. Martial arts and lifting can go well together, and the lifting will help the martial artist just like it will help any other athlete. Strength training will not make him better in the skills of the martial arts, but it will make him physically stronger and less likely to get injured.

I have several WST clients who are involved in the martial arts. I have a "Top 10 USA" kickboxer, a full-contact ultimate fighter, and several wrestlers and karate competitors. The regular guidelines of two whole-body workouts every seven to ten days apply the same to martial artists as to any other athlete. I would probably strive to make the strength-training workouts brief, under an hour, and focus on the core compound exercises for the whole body.

A stronger body will be beneficial to any athlete, including the martial artist, but to be better at *any* sport, skills must be improved, which lifting will not do.

BOB WHELAN'S Q&A

January 2004

Q. *I've become interested in the Hammer Pullover machine and want to acquire one for home use. What are your views on this machine?*

A. I'm a big advocate of the machine pullover, which has been called the *upper body squat.* It works most of the muscles in the upper body—lats, triceps, rear delts, pecs—so much so that it's hard to ignore using this machine if it's available. While some advanced and stronger-than-average lifters can perform the barbell pullover for variety, most will be limited by the strength of their triceps. With the machine version, this problem is minimized, and you also work over a greater range of motion with direct resistance.

I have the Hammer Pullover, and I use it with most of my clients. I incorporate a lot of partial forced reps, mostly for those under 5'10" tall, to get a smooth and complete range of motion over the last part of the concentric when bringing the crossbar all the way down to the waist. Trainees with longer-than-average torsos or upper-arm bones have better leverage on the machine and require less assistance from me. It doesn't only go by height, as I have some guys 6'5" and over who have a hard time with the machine because they have long legs and relatively short torsos.

To get maximum benefit from the machine, you shouldn't use so much weight that you can't drive the crossbar all the way down to your waist. You should have a one-second ("one-one thousand") pause at the point of the rep when the crossbar is near the waist. As with all exercises, good form is crucial for maximum results.

Q. *I've been reading lately about "round-back lifting," but I've also read that you should never lift with a rounded back. What's the deal? Is it a bad thing or just more risk involved?*

A. I would say that you're reading two different things here. Generally, for the vast majority of people and for the vast majority of the time, lifting with a founded back isn't a good thing. The general advice for most lifters who do most of the common strength-training exercises using conventional equipment is to keep the back flat rather than round.

Bob Peoples was a round-back-style lifter, but this was mainly due to his genetics—long arms and legs and short torso. Bob Hise II wrote that Peoples would approach the bar like most conventional deadlifters but would exhale instead of inhale before beginning the pull. He thought that this improved his leverage. He began with his legs, but they quickly straightened out and he was left with a long back pull. I believe that was due more to his unusually long arms than anything else. Long-armed lifters with short backs often have higher deadlifts than lifters of other proportions.

There's a form of advanced, specialized lifting—best avoided by most trainees—that intentionally uses a round back. This is needed for such things as odd-object lifting including stone lifting and Zerchers. It's an advanced way to lift specific items but not the way to lift weights as a general rule. While round-back lifting is something that most recreational lifters should avoid, some people naturally use it, such as grapplers, policemen, and firemen, who have to wrestle with a body or lift someone or something from the floor.

Q. *Is there evidence that explosive lifting leads to joint, tendon, back, or other problems as one ages? I'm the oldest lifter where I*

train and am always surrounded by high school kids lifting for their sports. Any thoughts?

A. There's a big difference between "explosive" and "ballistic." Lifting "heavy" usually involves moving the weight in a rapid, positive motion. I've trained using what could be called an explosive *concentric* motion for over 35 years with no real problems. I lower the weight slowly, so I wouldn't call it "ballistic" training. That's the key: to lower the weight slowly and under control.

There's no 100% right answer here. It's an individual thing, as you'll find examples of all sorts. Slower-speed training is good for those who have injury problems and for those who just enjoy it. I use slow-speed training too, and like it as a change of pace. I wouldn't worry about "exploding" on the concentric if you're lifting heavy. It's more of a frame of mind than the actual speed. With heavy weight for low to moderate reps, the weight will still move slowly up even if you think "explosive." That's the big difference between *explosive* and *ballistic*.

Ballistic lifting is usually done with a weight that's light, and it's moved quickly in both the positive and negative parts of the rep. some people advocate this but I don't, as I consider it dangerous. I can see nothing productive in lifting this way. I would focus mainly on good technique and lowering the weight slowly on the eccentric.

Q. *I've read that you recommend a multivitamin but not much else. Do you take supplements?*

A. Yes, but I'm conservative about recommending them. I view them as an "insurance policy" for health reasons only, *not* a phony way to get someone bigger and stronger faster. Only drugs do that.

The fitness industry is full of misinformation about supplements. I advise you to take *at least a good multivitamin-mineral tablet every day, and *do your own research on anything additional you may want to take for health reasons.

I take a good multi. I also take an 81 mg "baby aspirin" a day, a niacin supplement, and a few other things that I think are good *for me* with *my* family health history. If you have high cholesterol, you should check with your doctor, as niacin raises HDL dramatically and usually lowers total cholesterol numbers.

My mother recently went on a time released niacin regimen at the recommendation of her doctor. She uses time-release niacin, 500 mg in the morning and 500 mg at night. Her total numbers went from over 200 to 160 in three months! I take time released niacin, krill oil and a few other things for HEALTH.

If you're eating well and are healthy, you may not need supplements. Emphasis should always be on food, but the supplements fill the possible gaps of missing nutrients. A good vitamin-mineral pill each day is a wise move, a good insurance policy, and not a waste of money. As far as protein powder is concerned, you definitely don't need it in my opinion and can find more efficient and cheaper ways to get enough protein.

As I've said previously, if you need a protein supplement *in addition* to your three regular meals, I recommend lots of skim or 1% milk and/or two cans of tuna per day. With previous information about mercury in some fish—this caution goes back and forth every few years—you could use chicken or turkey instead of tuna. There's about 45 grams of protein in each can. You can also buy chicken breasts or fish fillets and cook them! I only said cans because I was a bachelor and I usually don't like to cook. I'm making it very simple.

A friend and client, Victor Peck, buys a giant bag of chicken breasts every week and cooks them all on Sunday. He separates them into daily portions so that he has his protein spaced out all week. You can find a way to get plenty of protein if you're determined.

Q. *It doesn't seem like many strongman competitors use HIT as* *you recommend in your articles. I think strongman competitions* *demonstrate strength at its best, so if HIT is the best, why isn't it* *being used?*

A. I used to like to say *high intensity training,* but when it got shortened to *HIT* and things began to be assumed about training due to that label, I began to dislike the label. What I use and teach is hard, heavy, *progressive strength training.* I don't use just HIT routines. I hate the term *HIT.* You *hit* in baseball or other bat-and-ball sports.

Don't jump to conclusions from the description of a routine in an article, done on a specific day, with a specific person. It depends on what that individual client is training for and is capable of.

If someone wants to compete in a strength sport where he demonstrates strength in a one-rep maximum, he must train using low reps and singles. Most trainees (and most of my clients) don't train for a strength sport, so, unless the article you read says the routine is for training a strongman competitor, don't assume that the routine would be recommended by me to train a strongman competitor.

I use all types of training—barbells, machines, fast reps, slow reps, high reps, low reps, to failure, and not to failure—depending on the client. What stays consistent is the balance of push and pull. I hate training labels. All methods can work if they are used *with* *progression.*

I'm not just an advocate of HIT. I'm a s*trength training advocate.* I was the NSCA DC State Director for five years, and the NSCA is pretty much the opposite of HIT.

I use a lot of the same stuff that HIT advocates use, but I use a lot of other stuff, too. That's why I hate labels. It's all just strength training to me.

Taking work sets to failure—a common component of HIT—is probably the most time-effective way to train, which is one reason why it's great for many if not most trainees.

Q. *I've read in your WST commandments and other writings that you're against doing isolation exercises. Don't you think that some* isolation exercises could be beneficial?

A. You read too much into what you think I wrote. I never said *not* to do *any* isolation exercises. In the commandments, I wrote that *the core* of your program should be the compound movements, not the isolation exercises. I've also said in other writings that some isolation exercises, when added to a program based on the compound exercises, can be productive. The key is that you're not *replacing* the compounds with the isolations.

As long as you're not looking for the easy way out by substituting the isolation exercises for the much harder multi-joint exercises, using a few isolation exercises *in addition* to your major compound exercises can be beneficial.

Q. When evaluating a client, how do you determine the amount of cardio training he or she should do, and what are some of your considerations?

A. I don't recommend the same cardio work for everyone. I

fluctuate my cardiovascular recommendations depending on the age, health, bodyfat percentage, and goals of the client. If the trainees are in their twenties and healthy but very thin and trying to gain weight, I may have them do no CV training to help them put on some muscle. If someone is preparing for a powerlifting contest, then the same thing—no CV work. For the vast majority of middle-aged individuals (who are probably not competing in a strength sport), a three-times-per-week program for 20 to 30 minutes duration each time is the bare minimum. What's the point of training? If health is an important issue, there should be no question about CV work. You must do CV training to train your heart. This is especially so for trainees who use very abbreviated strength-training routines that don't provide enough *overall* exercise.

The more of a problem that you have with bodyfat, the more CV training you should do. If you're fat and you're genetically inclined to remain so, you need to slowly and safely up the cardio to four or five days per week (of lower intensity) for about 45 minutes in duration to help keep the bodyfat under control. As you get into better shape, you can increase the intensity of the cardio workout and reduce its duration. The goal is to burn maximum calories as well as work the heart if you're trying to burn fat.

The *harder* you work with higher intensity, the more calories you'll burn in a given period. You must be in good enough shape to do this, though. Don't kill yourself trying to get into shape. As your condition improves, increase the intensity and shorten the duration. At first, though, just stay on the machine at a comfortable pace and build up your conditioning base. As far as it hurting your strength goes, so what if you lose ten pounds on your bench press? That's better than a heart attack! Once you get your bodyfat under control, then you can reduce the CV training to a more moderate frequency—from five to three times per week.

As I've noted previously, my opinion on cardio has changed somewhat over the last few years. The latest research shows that high-intensity or interval-type cardio is more beneficial than just a long moderate-intensity or comfortable workout. I now do shorter but more intensive cardio workouts. Work up to it gradually.

There's also a difference between training for performance and training for fitness. If you're doing your CV training for performance—if you're a marathoner or tri-athlete, for example—your strength training will suffer a lot. But if you're doing your CV training only for fitness, your strength will be affected far less, if at all. If you're strength training for strength performance, such as powerlifting, the CV training may hurt your performance. Most people are not training for performance, although they are competing with themselves to get stronger. They are training mainly for their own health and overall fitness.

You're born with a certain number of slow and fast twitch fibers, but the intermediate fibers (type 2a) can be converted and adapted to the type of training that you're doing. An extreme emphasis on cardio will convert a lot of these fibers to perform as if they were slow twitch.

Strength training will aid in fat loss. The harder you strength train, the more muscle you add, and as you get your bodyfat under control, you can decrease your CV volume and duration to a moderate level as your basal metabolic rate increases. Every pound of muscle tissue that you build will result in a passive burning of up to 25 to 30 calories per day. Over a period of time, the added lean muscle will be even more beneficial for weight control than the CV work. Ten additional pounds of lean muscle will result in a passive calorie expenditure of up to 250 to 300 calories per 24-hour period.

My CV recommendations also depend on the volume of your strength-training workouts. With the current trend of trying to find the minimum amount of training, you'll burn fewer calories. The shorter your strength-training workouts, the more cardio you need to do if your bodyfat is a problem—for the exercise *and* calorie burning.

348

BOB WHELAN'S Q&A

April 2004

Q. *What's the biggest single training-related mistake you've* made?

A. The first and most obvious mistake was overtraining, which I was guilty of for years. I still made progress because I was young and my recuperative powers were strong, but I trained four or more times per week for several years in my early twenties. (I usually trained four or five days per weeks, because I gave up on six very quickly.) I made the same mistakes that people now make, thinking that more training was more advanced and modern. I didn't realize, at the time, that people had been using split routines and bodypart routines for several decades already. Those routines just became a lot more popular as drug use came into the scene.

I was powerlifting at the time, and I remember that when I cut my training down from four or five split workouts to two whole-body workouts per week, my lifting total increased by well over 100 pounds in the following training year. The tired, worn-out feeling went away, I was enthusiastic about every workout, I had no aching joints any more, and I felt strong. I strongly urge you not to waste time on bodypart routines, *especially* ones that are more than four days per week. Without drugs, these programs simply don't work for most trainees and are a waste of time.

Q. *Who, past or present, has influenced you the most as far as your training knowledge goes, and why?*

A. I can't really mention any *one* person who stands out alone who has influenced my philosophy, but I can name a few who have greatly influenced me.

As a beginner first starting out, it was the combination of Bob Hoffman and John Grimek that first influenced me greatly through reading York's *Muscular Development* and *Strength and Health* magazines. They got me on the right track and got me to shift my focus from just fitness with bodyweight-only exercises to strength training with barbells. I'd been doing just bodyweight-only exercises from the age of ten. I got a barbell set on my thirteenth birthday, even though my father was against it and always warned me about getting "musclebound." I knew he was wrong, never listened to him about it, and just kept lifting. He was all for the push-ups and pull-ups, etc., and had the strong prejudice against barbells that was common in those days. Back then, most athletic coaches weren't in favor of barbells. How things have changed— now, all athletes lift, and any coach who dares say anything against strength training appears ignorant.

A few years later, in the late sixties, I was influenced by Bradley J. Steiner and read most of his great books and articles. I love his motivational style of writing, and I would always feel like training harder than ever after reading what he wrote.

I was strongly influenced by Peary Rader after I discovered *Iron Man* magazine in my late teens. It was Peary who planted the seeds in my brain to train only twice per week, although it took a few years of reading Peary "say it" before I finally started "doing it."

As I've gotten older, I've grown to appreciate the wisdom of Stuart McRobert, and I'm not just saying this because I wrote for *Hardgainer.* Stuart has taught me the importance of injury prevention. When you're young and feel indestructible, you may ignore and scoff at this advice, but when you get older and get a few injuries, you'll come around. It's definitely better to train safer, even what may seem overly safe, to avoid injuries. An injury can set you back for weeks, months, or years. And that's if it's not a serious injury. A *serious* injury can stop you from training permanently! I'm a lot more careful with my exercise selection now, and I hope to be able to train for another 50 years because of it.

Q. *Regarding the equipment you routinely use in your facility, which pieces do you value most and believe are of the most benefit to those you train?*

A. Since I believe in complete, whole-body, balanced training, I don't have one piece of equipment that I value most. If I had to have only one thing, it would be a barbell—a good Olympic set. Second, I would have a power rack. I'm glad I'm not forced to have just a power rack and barbell, though, because I believe I get a much better overall workout using all the stuff I have.

I'm an Iron Game and barbell guy at heart, but I also appreciate the great equipment we have available now that the old-timers didn't. my training philosophy is a combination of the best information from the old-timers mixed with the best modern information.

I was raised exclusively on free weights but now use a lot of the good quality plate-loaded machines, too. I don't just collect machines like some people do, and I don't really enjoy talking about machines. I don't believe that barbells are better or machines are better. They both work.

I believe that you should use the best tools you have available. If you have limited space or can only have limited equipment, you can't beat the barbell and power rack for overall bang for the training buck.

If you're lucky enough to have some of the great new machines, use them. But if you don't have them, don't fret—you don't really *need* them. You still have enough to get the job done, and done well, with a barbell and power rack.

As I've noted previously, for many years I trained only with York bars and plates and Jubinville gear. Just for me, this stuff was great; but for business, when I train ten people in a row, I can get exhausted because my job becomes more like that of a bricklayer because of all the plate changing and moving around of equipment. The Hammer Strength and Southern Xercise machines I now have are great and make my job a lot easier and generally safer for my clients, many of whom are middle-aged beginners.

The good machines are nothing more than "guided barbells"–just alternative tools to get the job done. They should be viewed as secondary to the work being done, not the reason for training success.

As I've written about it before, I had some of the best workouts of my life in crude, poorly equipped gyms. It's passion, effort, desire, and consistent hard training that makes even a simple barbell work wonders. You don't really need anything more.

At a small, dingy, minimally equipped gym at an air base in Germany, I had some of the best workouts of my life. The showers frequently had only cold water. The cables on the pulley machines were always broken. Someone was always painting something for an inspection. Even the barbell plates were painted several times during this period. They were black, gold, and white at different times. A few times they were still wet when we came to train, and we could smell paint fumes. We still lifted and got paint all over us. As long as there were bars and plates, we were happy! We rooted for each other. There was a lot of back slapping, screaming, yelling, grunting, groaning, and sweating. We had a sort of gang, and if someone wasn't there, we all knew it and would get on his case when we saw him at the chow hall. There was peer pressure to train.

The weight room was rundown, dark, damp, and cold; but to us, it was warm, bright, and full of energy and life. We loved that place! Weights were banging everywhere, and the too-few 10s, 5s, and 2-1/2 plates available were shared and tossed back and forth around the room. Everyone had chalk; in fact, it was all over us! We had a true brotherhood and so much fun training.

We would train no matter what the weather was, come sleet or snow. Even base alerts didn't stop us. We usually worked 24-hour shifts, but when a shift was over, we had free time. But we still had to comply with the "war game" conditions if we remained on the base. Most guys would get the hell out of the base after they ate and slept. We would bring our gas masks to the gym and still train. I can remember squatting in my gas mask.

We never missed workouts, grew like crazy, and made tremendous progress. Anyone who trained with us would have made at least as much progress as they ever had anywhere else (and probably more progress than ever). That we had only very basic equipment just didn't matter.

Q. *You've been training yourself and others for many years. What common trait have you noticed in individuals that indicates a high probability of training success?*

A. On average, the guys who are successful in strength training love to train. They don't miss workouts. They find a way to train. They don't make excuses why they can't train. They make do with the equipment they have available, not complain about which new machine they don't have. They don't just talk about training, read about it, or make excuses about why they can't do it. Instead, they lift–hard and regularly. These people are the backbone of the Iron Game. They are the passion and beauty of modern strength training. Their problems in training, if any, are usually related to overtraining, not laziness. I mean true overtraining, not the latest version of overtraining that used to mean just a regular, ordinary workout.

Many individuals now never train hard and still think they

overtrain. Their problem is that they need to *start* training hard and not micro-manage and constantly worry about how they think they overtrain. I have guys call me with a so-called overtraining problem. I ask them what they are doing, and after I hear it, I usually say, "Where's the rest of it?" Their workouts are often so short that I thought they gave me only part of it. They have no clue about overtraining and really don't like to train, which is the root cause of their problem.

The ones who succeed are usually just regular people who train with a tenacity and dedication that's anything but regular. They train because they love it. They believe in it. It's almost spiritual to them. They get no money, fame, or glory for it. No one is making them do it; they just do it for themselves. They would feel depressed if they couldn't do it. They love getting stronger and love to train hard and stretch their physical capacity to the limit. They live their lives by the code of our Iron Game forefathers and wouldn't dream of taking drugs, either. They are truly dedicated, and because they love it, it's not hard for them to be dedicated.

Trainees and clients who gain my respect earn it by doing. It's not just how much weight you lift that earns my respect. It's about the effort. Many beginners are not strong yet but will be later, but they work so hard that I'll respect them more than a lazy stronger guy. Those who are willing to put forth effort and dedication are the ones who earn respect and promote camaraderie and brotherhood. It's hard not to like a guy who works his ass off.

People who train hard themselves usually respect others who train hard. They respect hard work because they do it, too. They know how it feels. They understand how tough it is. It's frequently the person who doesn't train hard himself who fosters division and ill will and argues about minor training issues. You earn respect in strength training only by doing, not by talking. The "non-doing types" are those who sometimes spend hours each day on the Internet arguing about strength-training philosophy. They love to attack or put down others and hide behind a computer screen, usually thousands of miles away. Some of the PhD-researcher types fall into this category. They can talk forever about the physiological response to strength training, but they know nothing about real-world strength training because they don't do it themselves.

Serious trainees share a common goal and a common bond that unites us—passion for natural strength and hard training, and doing it ourselves. It's the true brotherhood of iron, strength, and hard work, and all are welcome if they are willing to pay the price of hard work and dedication. Race, religion, politics, or nationality don't matter when you're battling the iron. Citizenship to this "nation" requires only effort and doing, not excuses and theorizing.

"Train like a champion TODAY! ... Regular workouts are the best long-term investment *strategy."*

--Bob Whelan

Stuart McRobert's Hardgainer.com

Stuart McRobert has been publishing training information since 1989. Whether you're a bodybuilder, or a fitness or strength trainee, male or female, beginner or advanced, or want to train in a public gym or a home gym, he offers a WEALTH of information and wisdom. Regardless of your age or where you train, or whether you want to build a lot of muscle or just a little, you require training that's SAFE, PRACTICAL, and EFFECTIVE.

Stuart's qualifications for being able to help you: He's written five books on physique transformation. He's edited a training magazine, HARDGAINER, for 15 years.Since 1981 he's had over 400 articles on training published in newsstand magazines. He has over 30 years of personal experience of physical training.

He has a reputation for providing non-commercialized, honest instruction free of any association with the food supplement and exercise equipment industries. He also has a reputation for attention to detail, thoroughness, safety, and health that's rare in the training world. He's guided countless people with their training. He's studied training for over 30 years.

He is 100% against the use of steroids and PEDs.

He has many years experience of conferring with colleagues who are strength trainers, coaches, chiropractors, and researchers. And this process is ongoing.

All of CS Publishing's publications come with a money-back guarantee. If you're not fully satisfied with any of our printed publications, return what you bought within 60 days and you'll receive a no-questions-asked refund. There's no risk for you.

CS Publishing offers the best weight training books you will find on planet Earth; they are highly endorsed by Maximum Bob Whelan and Drew Israel, who both wrote many articles for Stuart's magazine *Hardgainer*. One of Stuart's books, *BRAWN*, is the first training book Bob Whelan recommends to his clients.

357

CYBERPUMP.com

Providing REAL Information on Various Aspects of the Weight Game - The CYBERPUMP.COM Network!

Cyberpump.com	IronHistory.com
IronHistoryArchives.com	BodyBuildingTube.com
StrengthMentor.com	TrainHardWithDrKen.com
ArthurJonesMuseum.com	GripBoard.com

MashMonster.com

Cyberpump! opened its doors on the web in 1995. Since then, they've been bringing you the real deal with respect to training information every day. Cyberpump! covers all aspects of training. From being THE resource for HIT to bodybuilding, strength training for sports, strongman, Iron History, and for meeting your individual training goals.

One of the biggest online library of articles covering training, nutrition, technique, and other aspects to build your physique. The most comprehensive library of articles on High Intensity Training.

The EXCLUSIVE republishing of the High Performance Newsletter articles. Some of the best content with respect to Hard Training published in the last decade!

A comprehensive Q&A section with over 10,000 Q&A's. Q&A writers with over 100 years of combined experience covering from all aspects of training. Writers such as Doug Daniels of PLUSA, Dr. Ken Leistner, Matt Brzycki, Stuart McRobert, Richard Winett, and many of the top strength coaches in the world.

Training logs you can reference that help motivate and inform you. Beginner's Corner - A comprehensive beginners section to get you started off on the right foot.

Iron History with Joe Roark. The most comprehensive online library on the history of the weight game. Updated every other week. Including Iron History Extras where old articles from past great publications are republished.

TotalCoaching: The Online Coaching Resource—TotalCoaching provides articles on physical and mental preparation from some of the top strength coaches in the world!

Cyberpump! also hosts one of the best forums on the web for training discussion: The Cyberpump! Iron Page. Hard training video clips, articles on strongman, and much, much more.

Bob Whelan's NaturalStrength.com

Olde-Time Physical Culture—Cutting Edge Exercise Science

NaturalStrength.Com has maintained a reputation as one of the most well informed, truthful, and introspective sites on the 'net since 1999.

NaturalStrength.com is an online think-tank, combining the best of the old with the best of the new, dedicated to truthful drug-free strength training information. Good articles about strength training, strength research, the harmful effects of steroids, the mental aspects of training, and irongame/physical culture history are always wanted.

Email articles to the editor: bobwhelan@naturalstrength.com

> "It seems to me that one of the greatest services that can be rendered by those of us who love the healthy activity of bodybuilding — as it was in the 1920's, 30's, 40's, 50's, and throughout most of the 1960's — when the goal was genuine strength, vigorous good health, and physical efficiency and fitness, is to do what YOUR SITE is doing; so POWER TO YOU, BROTHER!"
>
> --Bradley J. Steiner

Please visit NaturalStrength.Com

For Free Training Help Go To: NaturalStrength.Net

We discuss SERIOUS, DRUG-FREE, STRENGTH TRAINING. You must register to post. Just try to post and follow the cues. Your application will be approved asap and then you can post at will. It's FREE. Ask all the questions you want once registered.

We are honored to bring back the Physical Culture philosophy and keep it alive in the post-steroid era. Strength and good health are inseparable in our philosophy. We are united by our desire to maximize muscular strength and development without the use of performance-enhancing drugs.

Training hard and progressively without drugs is the bond that unites us.

QUALITY INFORMATION (not quantity of BS) is the goal of this board.

Please visit NaturalStrength.Net

WhelanStrengthTraining.com

WHELAN STRENGTH TRAINING
An Olde-Time Physical Culture Studio

Quality Personal Strength Coaching,
Instruction, Supervision, and Motivation

MAKING WASHINGTON, DC, STRONGER SINCE 1990

202-638-1708

There is something for everyone at WST!

Get stronger, build muscle, reduce your body fat, increase your lean body mass - strengthen bones, reduce your biological age.

WHY WAIT? Stay young and active - join WST today!

You always get full attention as all training is "one on one" and private. Top quality equipment in a great training environment, filled with olde-time Iron Game memorabilia. Home of positive motivation and eternal youth conveniently located downtown near Gallery Place Metro.

We are dedicated to helping you achieve your strength and fitness goals through your hard work under our guidance. We accept only those clients who are willing to make a serious commitment to their health and fitness. We require your commitment to working with us for three months. This is a conservative and realistic timeframe for you to achieve your health and fitness goals and to establish healthy habits that will last a lifetime.

For more information, please visit WhelanStrengthTraining.COM

For coaching by PHONE visit WhelanStrengthTraining.NET

Personal Coaching By Phone
with Bob Whelan

WhelanStrengthTraining.NET

WHELAN STRENGTH TRAINING:
FAMOUS OLDE TIME PHYSICAL CULTURE STUDIO

Now in our 21st Year!

Join the WST Family!

An invitation to be coached by Bob Whelan:

If you would like to access my coaching directly and have it tailored to suit your goals, please contact me regarding a telephone consultation. I'm here for you when you need me.

A single one-hour consultation could speed your progress and help you to reach your goals much sooner. Periodic follow-up consultations of a shorter duration would help to keep you on track and uncover other improvements to further your progress. Once I receive your order, I will email you with additional information, and we'll set up the time for the call.

Sign-up at WhelanStrengthTraining.NET

NaturalStrength Online Store

BobWhelan.com

We've Got What You Need!

* Strength Tools *
* Fitness Equipment *
* Nutrition *
*Martial Arts *
* Books *
* Music *
. . . and More!

We are an Amazon Store--

We've got what you need!

BobWhelan.com

The Best Personal Strength Coach in New York City

DrewIsrael.net

If you live in the New York City area and are looking for serious strength training, you must hire Drew "The Human Wall" Israel as your personal coach.

Drew is one of the most knowledgeable coaches in the field of strength training and is widely respected among his peers for his brute drug-free strength. He has 10,000 pounds of Olympic plates as well as every type of bar, bench, machine, and odd object you can imagine in his Queens facility.

If you want to take the next step and really get the results you deserve, contact Drew today.

Please visit DrewIsrael.net

MUSCLE SMOKE & MIRRORS
By Randy Roach

"An instant classic! I was blown away by its historical depth and quality of research. It is clearly one of the best Iron Game/Physical Culture history books ever written. This book sets a new standard for quality. Anyone even remotely interested in the weight game should get this book."

- Bob Whelan, M.S., C.S.C.S.

The research for this extensive, three volume project represents a comprehensive effort to establish a complete context from which the sport of bodybuilding arose. "Muscle, Smoke & Mirrors" is the rise and fall of what was truly once an extraordinary discipline associated with a term known as "Physical Culture." Experience what bodybuilding was originally and learn just exactly what Physical Culture really is. See what growing philanthropic power flexed its financial and political muscles to foster its corporate agenda, compromising human health internationally. Read how the merger of technology and politics culminated in the industrial-ization, commercialization, federalization, inter-nationalization and finally the STERILIZATION of a nation's food supply, rendering it suspect not only to the general public but also to the most elite of athletes. Whether you are a novice, an elite bodybuilder, or simply sports-nutrition minded, learn how the emerging forces of the Iron Game evolved. Ultimately, the factions of this industry would grow powerful and manipulative while fighting for control over the Game. It took the running of several parallel histories on body-building, nutrition, supplements and the role of drugs to offer a complete, first-time unraveling of the web of confusion and politics that still permeates the sport into the 21st century! Volume I of "Muscle, Smoke & Mirrors" is truly the untold stories surrounding "Bodybuilding's Amazing Nutritional Origins."

ORDER ONLINE AT:
RandyRoach.Ca
Coming 2011: Volume II, The Pumping Years...Nautilus Emerges!

366

To order more copies of this book please visit:

SuperNaturalStrength.com

To order copies of Bob's other book: *Iron Nation*, please visit:

IronNation.com

74520287R10219

Made in the USA
Middletown, DE
26 May 2018